Jogging and Walking
For Health and Fitness

Third Edition

Frank Rosato, Ed.D.
University of Memphis

Morton Publishing Company
925 W. Kenyon, Unit 12
Englewood, Colorado 80110

Printed in the United States of America

10   9   8   7   6   5   4

ISBN: 0-89582-295-4

Preface

The third edition of this text has been extensively revised. First and foremost, "walking" as a mode of exercise has been added. This is reflected in the title of this edition which now reads *Jogging and Walking for Health and Fitness*. Walking has been added because it: (1) is the natural form of locomotion for humans, (2) is becoming very popular as a fitness activity, (3) fits appropriately in the new ACSM guidelines for exercise, (4) is excellent for improving one's state of health, and (5) is versatile enough to be used as a lead-up for more vigorous forms of exercise, or it may be pursued vigorously so that it becomes the primary exercise.

Second, the fields of exercise science and health promotion are dynamic so that the pace of change is accelerating. What was considered to be an article of faith just 5 to 10 years ago may be discarded like a pair of worn out walking or jogging shoes today. In this edition, new information has replaced that which has become outdated, new trends have been identified, and the concepts and content that are presented are supported primarily by research that has been reported since the second edition was published.

Third, every chapter has been significantly affected in this revision. Also, there are eight chapters in this edition as opposed to the seven chapters in the second edition. Several of the chapter titles have been changed to better reflect their contents. The order of the chapters has been changed for a more logical presentation of the information.

The focus of this edition is consistent with that of its predecessors — the emphasis remains on the enhancement of health and fitness. The object is not to take novice exercisers and turn them into fierce competitors although the information in this edition and its intent does not preclude that. But the primary purpose is to take novice exercisers, introduce them to the benefits of walking and jogging, and present persuasive and logical reasons why they should take the time and make the effort to include exercise in their daily lives. The emphasis is to encourage ordinary Americans to start moving for health enhancement, or for improvement in physical appearance, or for the development of physical fitness, or for other reasons.

This edition provides the guidelines for novices to begin and sustain a walking or jogging program safely and effectively. The principles of exercise are presented, which appropriately applied by walkers and joggers, will result in the accomplishment of their health and fitness objectives. Also, veteran walkers and joggers may find information that is useful both for motivation and for refining established programs.

Nutrition is an important component of a healthy lifestyle and certainly important for active people. The latest nutritional concepts — the Food Guide Pyramid, new food labels for processed items, the antioxidant vitamins, etc. — are presented. The consistent application of sound nutritional concepts is beneficial to walkers and joggers as they attempt to achieve their objectives.

Guidelines and precautions for exercise in hot and cold weather are covered. Understanding the challenges imposed by both is the key to exercising effectively and safely in various environmental conditions. The prevention and treatment of common walking and running injuries are covered.

Finally, this edition is accompanied by an instructor's manual that should facilitate the preparation, delivery, and assessment of instructional and learning objectives. The Instructor's Manual includes learning objectives, chapter outlines (lecture outlines), and a test bank, consisting of true-false, multiple choice, definition, and short essay items. There are a total of 551 test questions that instructors may use to construct their tests. The Instructor's Manual will be made available to adopters of the book.

I would like to thank Ginger Lipsey, Kandra McBride, Anna Phalen, Sam Verzosa, Joseph Waade, Lisa Burkhardt, Karen Brown, and Jayesh Patel for allowing us to photograph them as they demonstrated the mechanics of walking and jogging and the techniques of stretching for both of these activities. I would also like to thank the staff at Morton Publishing Company for their patience and flexibility associated with deadlines as I prepared the manuscript. Thanks once again to Sheri Seiser for her excellent photographic work for this and other projects that we produced together. I wish to extend my gratitude to the managers of Q the Sports Club of Memphis for allowing us to take some of our photos at their excellent facility. Special thanks to Devonia Cage who, after putting in her regular day at work, took my handwritten manuscript home where she quickly turned it into a computer driven hard copy. Finally, I would like to thank my wife Pat for her patience and willingness to take on some of my responsibilities while I was involved in this project.

Frank Rosato, Ed.D.
Memphis State University

Contents

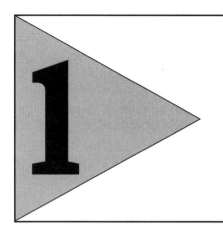

Physical Fitness in America

This chapter chronicles the current status of the physical fitness movement in America. Data generated from national polls and surveys have documented the extent of the movement and highlighted those segments of society that are heavily involved as well as those who are largely conspicuous by their absence. The latest exercise guidelines developed by The American College of Sports Medicine (ACSM) are presented here, as well as the reasoning behind the new approach.

The financial costs associated with sedentary living to an affected individual, along with the costs imposed on society for the consequences of such a lifestyle, are discussed. Fitness and wellness programs have been in existence long enough in the workplace that preliminary conclusions about their cost effectiveness are emerging. The early data are very encouraging for health care cost containment as well as other considerations that are important to the successful management of business.

The average workweek has expanded in the last ten years and, conversely, the hours available for leisure time have declined. It is becoming more difficult to find time for exercise, therefore time management skills and techniques are taking on more importance. Some time management tools are presented to assist users to find pockets of time that are available during the day for worthwhile pursuits such as exercise. Finally, a rationale is presented for choosing walking and/or jogging as safe and expeditious modes of activity for attaining physical fitness and health enhancement.

AMERICA ON THE MOVE

Throughout the United States, people can be seen walking, jogging, cycling, and swimming for the attainment of physical fitness, weight loss, and other health promoting reasons. Fitness clubs are packed with people doing aerobics to music or exercising with weights, stair-steppers, rowing machines, treadmills, and bikes. Newer and more sophisticated exercise equipment is being developed and marketed every day. Information regarding fitness and health appear in the print and electronic media daily.

The perception from this frenzy of activity is that most Americans are fully involved in the exercise movement. Unfortunately, perception and reality are not in agreement. Information gathered during the last 30 years indicates that the majority of Americans have never exercised enough to have a positive impact on their fitness level or their health status.

The current trend toward exercise began in the 1960s. During the early years, literally millions of sedentary people began exercising and the movement was growing rapidly. Eventually, the influx of new participants slowed down so that in the past few years a disturbing trend began to surface: The exercise movement has plateaued in spite of growth in the population.[1] This is occurring at a time when the health and wellness benefits associated with consistent participation in physical activities is most compelling. The American Heart Association (AHA) has recently recognized the importance of physical activity by declaring in 1992 that its opposite, physical inactivity, is a major risk for cardiovascular disease.[2] Further, the AHA has stated that, "Persons of all ages should include physical activity in a comprehensive program of health promotion and disease prevention."[3] In 1985, The American Cancer Society began recommending exercise to help people protect themselves from cancer.[4] The endorsements of exercise by prestigious but conservative organizations as these occurred because of the weight of research evidence. Considerable documentation was required for these organizations to make recommendations of this magnitude to the general public.

SURVEY RESULTS

A national survey in 1986 indicated that only one of every ten respondents exercised as frequently as four times per week.[5] The average frequency of participation was one time per week and 27% of the respondents never exercised. The same survey was administered in 1990 and the only significant change between it and the original one was that the average frequency of participation increased to one and one-half times per week.[6]

A survey by the National Sporting Goods Association indicated that the number of Americans who exercised at least twice per week increased from 30.8 million in 1987 to 32.2 million in 1989.[7] However, exercising two times per week falls short of the recommended amount needed to improve health and wellness. Even more disturbing is that 80% of the adults in this country do not exercise or do not exercise frequently enough.

In spite of overwhelming evidence that physical activity can reduce the incidence of chronic disease (heart disease, cancer, strokes, diabetes, osteoporosis, etc.) only 22% of adult Americans are exercising at the recommended level for health enhancement; 54% are barely active; and the remaining 24% are totally sedentary.

Physical inactivity is a risk factor that crosses all demographic boundaries. But the problem is worse for: (1) minority ethnic groups, (2) all people regardless of their ethnicity who are poorly educated, (3) older adults, and (4) those of lower socio-economic status. Unfortunately, chronic diseases are most prevalent in these population groups.

Physical inactivity is a risk factor that can be reversed easily and economically. The new recommendation for exercise developed by the American College of Sports Medicine for the purpose of health enhancement is that adults should accumulate at least 30 minutes of moderate physical activity over the course of most days (at least 4 days per week).[8] Scientific research has indicated quite clearly that compliance with this modest level of exercise can improve the health of individuals and, concomitantly, the health of the nation. Furthermore, exercise does not have to be structured or planned nor must it include the activities associated most with fitness and health such as jogging, cycling, rowing, swimming and the like. Vigorous exercises such as these provide the most benefit, but more moderate exercises including, but not limited to, everyday physical activities such as mowing the lawn (without a riding mower), gardening, raking leaves, walking, climbing stairs, and washing and waxing the car contribute to health promotion. Additionally, it is not necessary to exercise in a single continuous session. A total of 30 minutes of exercise sprinkled throughout the day is just as effective for health enhancement as one continuous bout. In other words, all activities that require physical exertion should be looked upon as opportunities for exercise and a bonus for health enhancement rather than chores that have to be done.

We can all benefit by adopting the philosophy that substituting our own muscle power for mechanically and electronically powered devices is an idea whose time is well past due. When possible, walk or bike instead of driving the car, climb stairs instead of using elevators and escalators, take a ten minute walk instead of a cup of coffee and a doughnut at breaktime, mow your own lawn instead of hiring someone else to do it, and wash your own car instead of running it through the car wash. By taking advantage of these and many other opportunities for physical activity you will surely meet the minimum criteria for health enhancement and you will look better and feel better as a result.

The first two editions of this text were concerned with jogging as the means for attaining fitness and health. This edition of the text has been expanded by the addition of "walking" in order to reflect the new guidelines for and attitude toward exercise. In a later chapter, you will be introduced to the benefits of walking for exercise and health.

FITNESS AND WELLNESS PROGRAMS IN BUSINESS AND INDUSTRY

Data that is accumulating from worksite fitness and wellness programs have provided more ammunition for the physically active life. Many of these programs have been in place long enough to have had an impact on employee health status. Companies that have invested in worksite health promotion programs are finding that they are saving more dollars than they spent initially as they attempt to contain the spiraling cost of health care.

It takes time and consistent effort for preventive practices to translate into changes in health status, and it takes an educational component to change long-standing behavior patterns such as cigarette smoking, poor nutritional practices, and sedentary living. It also takes time and a sincere commitment to control blood pressure and serum levels of cholesterol with lifestyle changes as opposed to medications.

The early data coming from worksite health promotion programs are very encouraging.

Companies are discovering that health care costs have been reduced, there is less worker absenteeism, greater employee productivity, and fewer on-the-job accidents.[9] Health promotion programs with physical fitness opportunities either on site or paid for (partially or fully) by the company is a perk that has been used to recruit and keep key personnel.

The initial capital outlay for establishing a comprehensive worksite health promotion program can usually be recovered in two to three years.[10] The potential company savings from reduced medical costs, reduced absenteeism, increased productivity, and decreased worker turnover is in the range of $2 to $6 for every dollar invested.

THE FINANCIAL PRICE TAG FOR SEDENTARY LIVING

Many studies have shown that exercise of moderate intensity that is performed consistently reduces all-cause mortality and delays or reduces the likelihood of incurring chronic diseases.[11,12,13] An active lifestyle benefits those who are active as well as those who are not.[14] First, active people place less demand on the nation's medical delivery system, and second, they are more productive occupationally. Conversely, those who choose to lead sedentary lives impose the costs associated with their lifestyle on others.

The cost to others (referred to as "external costs") by those who are physically inactive are due to additional payments received by them primarily from collectively financed programs such as health insurance, sick-leave payments, disability insurance, and group life insurance. Active people pay the same premiums and payroll taxes to finance these programs as the sedentary people who are the most frequent users. The limitation of these programs is that they do not distinguish utilization frequency

nor do they provide discounts for health behaviors, therefore they function as social welfare programs that subsidize unhealthy behaviors.

Everyone benefits when sedentary people gravitate to an active way of life. Each minute that people spend walking increases life expectancy by one minute.[15] Since joggers burn calories twice as fast, they can expect a return of double their exercise time in life expectancy. The Rand Corporation, the well-known California based "Think Tank" has developed a theoretical model that projects the following: each mile that a sedentary person walks or jogs will add 21 minutes to that person's life and save society 24 cents in medical and other costs. The economic drain of sedentary living on society is double the external cost associated with cigarette smoking.

CONTRIBUTING TO THE PROBLEM

The fitness movement was largely a reaction to developments in medicine, science, and technology and their relationship to the changing disease and death patterns in the nation. Communicable diseases (tuberculosis, pneumonia, typhoid fever, smallpox, scarlet fever, etc.) were the leading causes of death during the early years of this century. Advances in medical science have virtually eradicated these maladies and threats to life, but they have been replaced by chronic degenerative diseases such as heart disease, stroke, cancer, diabetes, etc. This group of diseases is largely lifestyle-induced and has reached epidemic proportions. Many authorities refer to these chronic diseases as voluntary or self-inflicted. This emphasizes the influence of negative choices and unhealthy behaviors on the development and course of these diseases.

Cardiovascular disease accounts for approximately 44% of all deaths in the United States.

Approximately 69,080,000 Americans have one or more forms of cardiovascular disease.[16] Cardiovascular diseases are responsible for 950,000 deaths annually with about one-half of these (500,000) the result of coronary heart disease. This is the type of heart disease that most Americans are aware of, but most of them don't fully understand the behaviors that are needed to prevent or delay it. The Framingham Heart Study — a landmark study of heart disease — identified the risk factors connected with heart disease. This ongoing study began in 1949 and continues to this day turning out valuable information from the subjects they began studying decades ago.

As risk factors were identified there evolved the realization that heart disease was not the inevitable consequences of aging but an acquired disease that was potentially preventable. Cigarette smoking, high blood pressure, elevated levels of blood fats, diabetes, overweight, stress, lack of exercise, and a family history of heart disease were found to be highly related to heart attack and stroke. Fortunately, most of these risk factors can be modified by the way we live.

We have within our control the opportunity and the right to choose what to eat and how much, whether or not to smoke cigarettes, whether or not to exercise and how we control stress. We can choose when to be screened for blood pressure and blood fats and we can choose whether or not to act upon that information. During the last four decades, millions of Americans have changed eating, smoking, and exercise habits and, consequently, deaths from cardiovascular disease declined by approximately 51% during this time.[17] Other factors are involved in this favorable trend, but modifications in lifestyle have made their contribution.

Our lives today are considerably different from life in the early years of this century.

Scientific and technological advances have made us functionally mechanized. Labor saving devices proliferate all phases of life — our occupations, home life, and leisure time pursuits — always with the promise of more and better to come. Each new invention helped foster a receptive attitude toward a life of ease and we have become accustomed to the easy way of doing things. The mechanized way is generally the most expedient way and in our time-oriented society, this became another stimulus for us to indulge in the sedentary life.

Today, exercise for fitness is contrived; it is programmed into our lives as an entity separate from our other functions. On the other hand, the energy expenditures of our forefathers was integrated into their work, play, and home life. Physical fitness was a necessary commodity and fit people were the rule rather than the exception. Tilling the soil, digging ditches and working in factories were physically demanding jobs. Lumberjack contests and square dances were vigorous leisure pursuits. Being a wife and taking care of home and family required long hours at arduous tasks. In the early years of this century, one-third of the energy for operating the factories came from muscle power. By 1970, this figure dropped to less than one percent and is reflective of the declining energy demand of our jobs.

The turn of the century found 70% of the population working long, hard hours in the production of food. Children of this era walked several miles to school and did chores when they returned home. Today, only 3% of the population, using highly mechanized equipment, are involved in the production of food, and their children ride to school. Adults drive to the store, circle the parking lot to get as close as possible to the entrance and ride elevators and escalators while there. We mow the lawn with a riding mower, play golf in a cart, wash dishes and clothes in appropriate appliances, change television channels with a remote control, and open garage doors in the same manner.

These are simply observations of life in America and are not intended to imply that the fruits of science and technology are repudiated, but rather that their results, along with their impact upon us, be viewed in perspective and acted upon accordingly. Mechanization has reached our leisure time and it is in this sphere that we must commit some time to vigorous activity because it has been effectively removed from other areas of life. Mechanization permeates all facets of our lives.

Decades ago, futurists predicted that Americans would be working a four-day workweek of about 32 to 34 hours. The promise of extended leisure time was attractive to America's workforce. But, the futurists were wrong. The workweek has not decreased, in fact, quite the opposite has occurred.[18] The workweek is the longest it has been since the mid 1950s. Americans had 26.2 hours per week of leisure time in 1973. By 1989, this dropped to 16.6 hours per week.[19] The average workweek in 1976 was 40.6 hours, but by 1989 it had increased to 46.8 hours.

This trend has increased the difficulty of finding a time to schedule exercise. Effective management of time is becoming more important as we attempt to balance work, leisure activity, and sleep in a 24 hour day. To commit the time and effort required to exercise consistently, one must understand its relevance for a healthy life.

TIPS FOR MANAGING TIME

Effective time managers are skilled in identifying and prioritizing their goals. They identify the ultimate objective and then set realistic short-term goals that are attainable with sustained effort. The goals that are established should be quite specific so that progress can be evaluated. Lastly, goals should be accompanied by a time-line for their accomplishments.

Effective time managers use a variety of tools to help them accomplish their daily tasks. For example, many people generate a "list of things to do for today." This is carried on their person on a 3 x 5 index card or pocket size notebook. The tasks are crossed off as they are completed during the day.

Another tool features the development of a weekly or monthly calendar. The calendar should contain the fixed items that occur every week such as classes, work, meals, and meetings. Also to be included are important non-fixed items such as tests, due dates for written and oral assignments, and vacation. The completion of such a calendar will indicate pockets of time that are available for physical activity, study, and other pursuits. You will be surprised how much time is left over from these activities when total time is systematically examined in this manner.

As important as time availability is, individuals still must be motivated to use it constructively. A national survey conducted among "less active" Americans indicated that 84% of them watched television a minimum of three hours per week.[20] This suggests that they have leisure time available but that they would rather watch television than participate in physical activity.

RATIONALE FOR CHOOSING WALKING AND JOGGING AS THE MODE OF ACTIVITY

Man has inhabited the earth for many centuries but only the last seventy-five years have generated such drastic changes in lifestyle. Our basic need for physical activity has not changed. Our bodies were constructed for, and thrive, on physical work but we find ourselves thrust into the automobile, television, and sofa age and we simply have not had enough time to adapt to this new sedentary way of living. Perhaps 100,000 years from now the sedentary life will be the healthy life. But at this stage of our development, the law of use and disuse continues to work. That which is used becomes stronger and that which is not used becomes weaker. For simple verification of this physiological principle, just witness the results of a leg in a cast for eight weeks and note the atrophy that has occurred to the limb during that time.

It is the belief of many people, this author included, that our new ways of living are precipitating or at least significantly contributing to the diseases that are affecting modern affluent man. They are unique to the highly industrialized nations. By contrast, the underdeveloped nations, with their different lifestyles, do not experience this phenomenon to the same extent.

Before developing and/or engaging in any form of physical exercise, beginners should determine what their expectations are from exercise. In other words, what are the goals, both short- and long-term they wish to achieve? Goal identification provides guidance regarding how hard, how often, how long, and what activities should be employed in the exercise program. Once these questions are resolved, the program can be tailored to meet the exerciser's specific objectives and if individuals follow through, there will be a high probability of success.

The choice to walk, jog, or to combine both as the activity mode by which one's health and fitness objectives can be attained has a significant base of support in the research literature. Both activities are effective and popular.

Walking

Walking is the natural form of locomotion for human beings. It is a low risk, low impact activity that can be done almost anywhere, by almost anybody (including many who are disabled), in most environments, and at some reasonable speed.

Walking uses a heel-to-toe motion so that the foot strike at landing occurs at the heel and the push off occurs at the end of the big toe. This action dissipates the force of impact with the ground over the widest possible foot area. As the foot rolls forward, horizontal momentum is generated for forward movement. The advancing foot lands before the rear foot leaves the ground insuring that one foot is always in contact with the ground. Forward motion of this type minimizes the impact of landing.

Walking is an effective way to introduce beginners to physical activity. Walking can be manipulated to meet a variety of objectives. In addition to being an entry point into exercise, it can be a lead-up conditioner for other types of activity. Or, it can be the end product for developing and maintaining physical fitness. This can be accomplished through brisk walking, or variations such as speed walking, power walking, and race walking.

Millions of people are walking for health and fitness. There are more than 10,000 walking events held annually. These include walk-a-thons, fun walks, and competitive race walks. There are more than 6500 walking clubs scattered throughout the country. Some of these include and/or feature hiking and orienteering (using a map and compass to find the path between two land marks).

Slow walking speeds produce substantial health benefits but result in a minimal increase in fitness level. Higher speeds result in improvements in both health and fitness. In a recent study, women subjects were divided into three groups of different walking intensity.[21] One group walked at 3 mph (strollers), a second group walked at 4 mph (brisk walkers), and the last group walked at 5 mph (aerobic walkers). The subjects walked three miles per day, 5 days per week. At the end of 24 weeks the data were analyzed. The results indicated that physical fitness improved on a dose-response basis, that is, the fastest walking group improved the most while the slowest walking group improved the least. But, the risk of cardiovascular disease reduced equally among the three groups. The 3 mph walkers benefited as much as the fastest walkers with regard to favorably changing the cardiovascular risk profile. If health enhancement is one's major exercise objective, walking — even slow walking — fits the bill nicely. If however, one's major objective is to improve physical fitness, fast walking is a very satisfactory activity. The bonus for those who engage in exercise for the purpose of fitness is that they achieve the health benefits simultaneously.

Jogging

Compared to walking, jogging is a higher impact activity. Jogging requires that both feet must be off the ground for a split-second during every stride. Since joggers become airborne, their impact with the ground is greater and the expenditure of energy is higher than that of walking except under two circumstances. First, the energy expenditure or oxygen cost of very slow jogging (5 mph) is equal to walking at the same speed. At speeds greater than 5 mph, the oxygen cost of walking exceeds that of jogging due to the inefficiency associated with very fast walking. Second, the oxygen cost of jogging up a hill is about one-half that of walking up the same hill. Since both feet come off the ground during jogging,

some of the vertical lift needed to run up the hill occurs naturally thereby lowering the net cost of the vertical work.

Although some surfaces are better than others, jogging is an activity that can be pursued almost anywhere that is devoid of hazards such as potholes or jutting rocks. It is also time-effective. For instance, it may take one hour to walk four miles but only 35 to 40 minutes to slow-jog the same distance. The savings in time is important to many busy people.

In spite of the fact that jogging has declined somewhat in popularity in the last few years, it nonetheless remains alive and kicking. It is estimated that there are 25 million people who jog a minimum of three times per week. Studies have shown that joggers are very dedicated to this activity and they are very compliant exercisers. Jogging will always be an effective means of improving health and fitness and it should continue to appeal to a large number of participants.

Other factors contribute to the appeal of walking and jogging. Both activities can be performed either indoors or outdoors and in most environmental conditions. From the perspective of equipment needs, a good pair of walking shoes for walkers and a good pair of jogging shoes for joggers is mandatory for protection against potential injury. The environmental conditions in which either is practiced should dictate the remainder of the attire.

Another appealing factor is that participants may walk or jog alone or with others. Walking or jogging in solitude provides the opportunity for introspection, or to mentally organize that paper that you must write for class, or it provides a setting for the mind to roam freely. Walking or jogging also provides the opportunity for socialization and camaraderie with friends who are similarly interested in exercise and it is a natural setting for a discussion of training programs, objectives and goals, training problems, nutritional habits, etc. Participation with others also provides motivation, a sense of competition and cooperation, and a commitment not to skip the next workout.

JOGGING AND WALKING FOR HEALTH AND FITNESS

The primary purpose of health-related exercise is the prevention of disease and the attainment of well-being. This can be achieved by consistent participation in mild to moderately vigorous aerobic activities. The components of health-related fitness are (1) cardiorespiratory endurance, which is the maximum ability to take in, deliver, and extract oxygen for physical work, (2) muscular strength, which is the maximum amount of force that a muscle or group of muscles can exert in a single contraction, (3) muscle endurance, which is the capacity to exert repetitive muscular force, (4) flexibility, which is the range of movement around the joints of the body, and (5) body composition, which is the amount of fat versus lean tissue in the body.

The accomplishment of aerobic physical fitness requires individuals to exercise vigorously enough to improve cardiorespiratory endurance and muscle endurance. Exercises for the development and maintenance of physical fitness increase the energy level and enhance physical appearance. A high degree of aerobic fitness may be developed by exercising five days per week, for approximately 45 minutes per exercise session, at an intensity level of 70% to 80% of the maximum heart rate

EXERCISE FOR PERFORMANCE

Performance-related fitness requires the abilities necessary for the proficient execution of sports skills. These abilities are not necessary for health enhancement but they are indispensable for those who participate competitively in physical activities. Speed, power, balance, coordination, agility, and reaction time are the performance-related components. Successful performance in games such as racquetball, tennis, basketball, volleyball, badminton, to name but a few, is dependent upon the possession and refinement of these athletic abilities. On the other hand walking, jogging, stationary cycling, stair stepping devices, and rowing machines require minimum amounts of athletic ability. These can be performed by most people. But the health-related and performance-related components are not mutually exclusive. Some individuals prefer to perform in athletic contests as the means by which they meet their health-related goals. Conversely, a competitor in endurance type events is developing the health-related components even though the major goal is performance-related. The idea is that the perceived lack of athleticism should not be a barrier to exercise for health enhancement because there are many health-related activities that require very little athletic ability.

Summary

▶ Survey data indicated that most Americans do not exercise often enough or vigorously enough to improve their health status.

▶ The exercise movement has plateaued in the last few years, in spite of compelling evidence that exercise is necessary for health and wellness.

▶ The American Heart Association has classified physical inactivity as a major risk factor for heart disease.

▶ Only 22% of American adults are exercising at the level recommended for heart health.

▶ Physical inactivity is more prevalent among (1) minority groups, (2) the poorly educated, (3) older adults, and (4) those who are in the lower socio-economic levels.

▶ For health enhancement, the American College of Sports Medicine recommends participation in mild to moderate physical activity over the course of most days.

▶ Everyday activities such as walking, stair-climbing, mowing the lawn, raking leaves and similar activities contribute to health and wellness.

▶ Exercise does not have to occur in one continuous bout; it can be divided up during the day.

▶ Fitness and wellness worksite programs are cutting the cost of health care due to less absenteeism, greater productivity and fewer on-the-job accidents.

▶ Consistent exercise participation reduces the risk of all-cause mortality.

▶ Those who follow a sedentary lifestyle receive more payments from health insurance, disability insurance, group life insurance, and take more sick leave than physically active people.

▶ The Rand Corporation estimated that each mile that a sedentary person walks or jogs will add 21 minutes to that person's life and save society 24 cents in medical and other costs.

▶ The risk factors for heart disease were identified by researchers who participated in the Framingham Study.

▶ The death rate from cardiovascular disease declined by 51% in the last four decades.

▶ Mechanization, the product of science and technology, has removed much of the labor from our occupations, homes, and leisure time activities.

▶ The workweek has been on the increase during the decades of the eighties and nineties.

▶ As leisure time decreases, time management skills assume greater importance as we attempt to balance work and play.

▶ Time management techniques are available to help us organize our time.

▶ Walking for exercise is a low risk, low impact activity that can be performed in most environments at some reasonable speed.

▶ Walking is a versatile exercise that can satisfy the needs of beginners or experienced exercisers.

▶ Walking can enhance health and/or develop aerobic fitness.

> Jogging is a higher impact activity when compared to walking but it burns more energy and uses more oxygen under most conditions.

> At approximately 5 mph, the oxygen cost of walking is equal to that of jogging.

> Walking up hills requires more oxygen than jogging up the same hills.

> Walking and jogging are inexpensive forms of exercise that can be performed indoors or outdoors.

> A quality pair of walking shoes for walkers and a quality pair of jogging shoes for joggers are important to prevent potential injury.

> Walking and jogging contribute to the health-related fitness components of cardiorespiratory endurance, flexibility, and body composition.

> The components of performance-related fitness include speed, power, coordination, agility, balance, and reaction time.

REFERENCES

1. Statement of American College of Sports Medicine "Prevention and President Clinton's Health Care Reform Proposal," Presented by S. P. Van Camp to the Subcommittee on Health; Committee on Ways and Means; U.S. House of Representatives, Oct 26, 1993.

2. "It's Official: Inactivity Increases Coronary Risks." *Harvard Health Letter*, 3, No. 3: Nov., 1992, p. 8.

3. "It's Official: Inactivity Increases Coronary Risks."

4. American Cancer Society. *Cancer Facts and Figures 1992*, Atlanta, GA: American Cancer Society, 1992.

5. *Sports Illustrated*. "Sports Poll 86" Time, Inc., 1986.

6. "Sports Illustrated on Sports." *ARAPCA Newsletter*, XII, No. 2: Winter, 1992, p. 12.

7. "Exercise Boom Continues." *ARAPCA Newsletter*, XII, No. 2: Winter, 1991, p. 8.

8. "An Easy-to-Swallow Prescription," *University of California at Berkeley Wellness Letter*, 10, Issue 2: Nov. 1993, p. 6.

9. Berters, R. "The Effects of Workplace Health Promotion on Absenteeism and Employment Costs In a Large Industrial Population," *The American Journal of Public Health*, 22, No. 8: July 1, 1991, p. 68.

10. Feineman, N. "From Boardroom to Locker Room: A Look at the 10 Year Metamorphosis of Corporate Fitness Plans," *Health*, 22, No. 8: Sept, 1990, p. 49.

11. Blair, S. N. et al. "Physical Fitness and All-Cause Mortality — A Prospective Study of Healthy Men and Women," *Journal of the American Medical Association*, 262, No. 17: Nov, 3, 1989, p. 2395.

12. Paffenbarger, R. S. et al. "The Association of Changes In Physical Activity Level and Other Lifestyle Characteristics With Mortality Among Men," *The New England Journal of Medicine*, 328, No. 8: Feb. 25, 1993, p. 538.

13. Duncan, J. J. et al. "Women Walking For Health and Fitness," *Journal of the American Medical Association*, 266: 1991, p. 3295.

14. Keeler, E. B. et al. "The External Costs of a Sedentary Lifestyle," *American Journal of Public Health*, 79: 1989, p. 975.

15. Keeler, "The External Costs of a Sedentary Lifestyle."

16. American Heart Association. *1992 Heart and Stroke Facts*, Dallas, TX: American Heart Association, 1991.

17. American Heart Association, *1992 Heart and Stroke Facts*.

18. Liscio, J. "America Is Going Back To Work Again," *U.S. News World Report*, May 11, 1992, p. 55.

19. Hales, D. *Your Health*, Redwood City, CA: Benjamin Cummings, 1991.

20. "Most Less Active Americans Want to be More Active," *NASPE News*, Winter, 1994, p. 11.

21. Duncan, J. J. et al. "Women Walking For Health and Fitness," *Journal of The American Medical Association*, 266: 1991, p. 3295.

2

Motivation and Motivational Techniques: Stimulants for the Physically Active Life

This chapter explores the challenge of motivating people to begin and maintain an active way of life. This is a formidable and perplexing task. Although much has been said and written about the value of exercise, only 22% of Americans are active enough to improve their health status. Even though we are 30 years into the current exercise movement, the majority of Americans are essentially sedentary. Either they are not convinced of the value of exercise, or they are unaware of its value, or they would rather be sedentary regardless.

Motivating people to begin exercising is indeed difficult, but it is even more difficult to keep them in compliance once they begin. The exercise dropout rate is 50% during the initial six months,[1] and the majority of these discontinue their exercise programs during the first three months.[2] It is ironic that most of the fitness benefits achieved by previously sedentary people occur during the first couple of months of training, yet the dropout rate is high during this time.

The reason most often advanced for not exercising by the "least active" Americans is that they don't have enough time.[3] Most often, this can be translated to mean that exercise is low on their list of priorities so it is usually squeezed-out of the daily schedule in favor of more preferred endeavors. Other barriers to exercise include inconvenient or inaccessible exercise location, work conflicts, poor spousal support, and occupational travel requirements.

13

BASICS OF MOTIVATION

Motivation is a label invented by people to describe a characteristic type of behavior. It cannot be measured directly; therefore it is inferred through observations of behaviors and actions. Such imprecision often results in inaccurate perceptions about presumed levels of motivation. The matter is confused further because motivation, as with other aspects of human behavior, lacks a uniformly acceptable definition. For this text, we will adopt the following definition: Motivation is any state or condition that causes an organism to produce or inhibit an action or motor response.[4] This is an expansive definition that includes both the internal and external forces that stimulate and affect behavior.

External forces, including external (extrinsic) rewards are important and necessary sources of stimulation that encourage novice exercisers to initiate and continue their exercise adventures. External rewards may be (1) symbolic: a badge, pin, or T-shirt; (2) material: money, prizes, payment for fitness club membership or dues; and (3) psychological: attention, recognition, and encouragement. While rewards of this type are initially important, the motivation that sustains exercise behavior is internal or intrinsic. Internal motivators of exercise behavior include the sense of accomplishment and satisfaction that one receives from participation, the value inherent in the activity to the participant, and the amount of fun and enjoyment derived.

Human behavior is purposeful; that is, it is goal-directed. The objective of motivated behavior is the achievement of our goals. Positive reinforcements (intrinsic as the base to build upon supplemented judicially with extrinsic reinforcements) motivate us to persist in the attainment of our goals. A workable plan for achieving goals involves knowing what we want to accomplish in the long run. In other words, we should be able to identify our long-range goals. Then we should set realistic short-term goals that may be reached within a reasonable time. The achievement of each short-term goal acts as both a reinforcer and a stimulus motivating us to strive for the next goal, while each accomplishment brings us closer to realizing our long-term goal. The key is realism: setting goals that are difficult enough to provide a challenge but yet have a reasonable chance for achievement. This is a feasible way to approach your fitness goals.

Some psychologists have determined that a moderate level of motivation is optimal. Too little is likely to result in early failure and too much may result in injury and burnout. In either case, motivation is adversely affected, adherence wanes, and the program, with all its good intentions and potential benefits, is terminated. This is graphically depicted by the Inverted U Hypothesis that appears in Figure 2.1.

In order to avert this all-too-familiar scenario, we must cultivate the philosophy that our health and fitness goals should be approached slowly and patiently, albeit progressively. We must learn to contain our enthusiasm so as not to attempt too much too soon during the early phases of the program. Remember, physical fitness is not achieved with only two weeks of training. The development and maintenance of physical fitness should be a life-long affair. This requires a sizeable commitment of time and knowledgeable effort, but the results are eminently worthwhile. You supply the time and effort and this text will provide you with the necessary knowledge. The appropriate application of these ingredients will increase your likelihood of success.

Factors that are motivating to one person may not have the same effect upon another due to differences in experience, interests, aims,

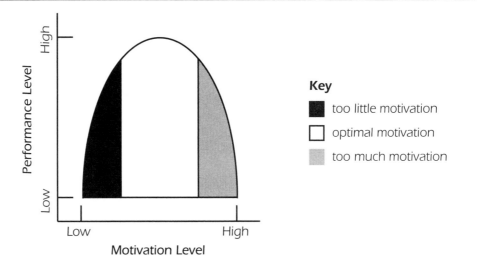

Figure 2.1 The Inverted U Hypothesis.

objectives, intelligence, etc.; therefore, selection of the exact factor or factors that will motivate any given individual to participate in a long-term walking or jogging program is conjectural at best.

Most people become involved with exercise for health-related reasons. These include weight loss, reduction of stress and anxiety, prevention or delay of heart disease, strengthening the musculoskeletal system, desire to live better and longer, and to sleep more restfully. The original reason for participation often becomes the primary reinforcer for maintaining the program. In some instances the original reason is blended with others or assumes lesser importance as progress occurs and new goals assume greater priority.

Unfortunately, being knowledgeable about the beneficial health effects of exercise is usually not enough of a motivator for many people. Most people know that exercise is good for health enhancement yet the majority of them don't participate. Having some knowledge simply is not enough to stimulate people

to make positive lifestyle behavioral changes. Millions of people know that smoking cigarettes is harmful to their health yet they continue to smoke.

It is difficult to determine which event or set of circumstances will motivate a given individual. We have at our disposal a variety of techniques that may enhance exercise continuance. These help, in a general way, to maintain the enthusiasm for a physically active life. However, predicting the precise motive that will stimulate a specific individual to exercise remains elusive. The following strategies may help.

 SOME MOTIVATIONAL STRATEGIES

Develop a Knowledge Base

Understanding the need for exercise as well as the associated health-related benefits may be a sufficient stimulus for some people to act but it is inadequate for the majority of sedentary individuals. However, Ken Cooper's first book motivated millions of sedentary Americans to become physically active. Knowledge provides a rationale for an active life, and for those who respond positively to cognitive information, it may be a primary motivator. As such, it should not be deleted from the techniques which are commonly employed to enhance exercise adherence.

Set Realistic Goals

Set realistic goals for exercise that are specific and attainable. These should address the major accomplishments that you will attempt to achieve. Your goals may include such factors as weight control, muscle development, an increase in energy reserves, management of stress, reductions in serum cholesterol and/or blood pressure, prevention of chronic disease, and competition in road races. Walking and jogging, or a combination of the two, are effective exercise modalities for achieving all of these goals.

Novice walkers may walk for 20 to 30 minutes per day, four to five days per week. Beginning joggers should jog for 20 minutes per day three times per week. This does not include the time required for warming up and cooling down. Beginners should ease into jogging by combining it with walking in order to diminish the musculoskeletal and cardiorespiratory stress. As the level of fitness improves, walking time should be reduced while jogging time progressively increases to fill the entire 20 minutes. There should be no increase in speed during this time. Jogging every other day will result in enough rest between exercise sessions for full recovery to occur.

As fitness improves, walkers may exercise more often (frequency) and for a longer period of time (duration). Since walking is a low impact activity, it imposes less demand upon the musculoskeletal system than does jogging. However, the intensity of walking should reflect a pace that is well-tolerated so that recovery may occur from one workout to the next. Reasonable exercise and health goals should be selected within these parameters.

Be patient — do not attempt nor expect too much too soon. Exercising beyond your capacity will produce pain, discomfort, and may possibly lead to injury. The occurrence of any or all of these events is likely to lead to discouragement, and ultimately to dropping out.

Select the Social Contexts That Are Most Supportive

People can choose where and with whom they will exercise. Whether to workout alone or with others is dependent upon one's preference, personality, exercise needs and goals, and compatibility with other exercisers. There is evidence to support both approaches and there are advantages associated with both. Some people prefer primarily one or the other, while others employ both in the attainment of their exercise goals.

Attractive features of the group approach include camaraderie, the possibility of developing productive social relationships with other group members, cooperation, competition, and reinforcement. The social support received from the group, particularly during the early weeks of a beginner's program, enhances compliance and this is the best approach for them.[5] Other people find that the individual approach to exercise is best for them. A one-year study of older men and women showed that an individual home-based exercise program was more effective than a group program in promoting exercise adherence.[6] The researchers found that the group exercise program proved to be too inconvenient over the course of one year. Convenience and accessibility of the exercise facility were important considerations that affected adherence to the group program. Unless these two factors are satisfactorily resolved, the independent approach might be best.

Exercise with a Buddy

Two people with similar training routines and compatible levels of physical fitness can provide motivational support for each other. Buddies can motivate each other, they can share their knowledge about fitness training, nutrition, and a host of other subjects of common interest to them. A bonus of the buddy system is that it becomes more difficult to skip a workout, even when you would rather do something else, when someone is waiting for you at a designated time and place.

Enlist the Support of Those Who Are Important to You

Spouses, other family members, friends, and co-workers — those with whom you frequently interact and whose advice you value — can be important sources of motivation, encouragement, and reinforcement. These respected people can provide support by projecting a favorable attitude toward your newly acquired exercise behavior. A number of studies have shown that spousal support is particularly influential.

The support received from others is more effective when they are themselves exercisers. As such, they function as role models who can draw upon their knowledge and experiences to assist, and to provide counsel and advice to you. It also helps if they will occasionally work-out with you.

Associate with Other Exercisers

Associate with other exercisers who motivate you in positive ways regarding physical activity. Catch their enthusiasm and give them some of yours. Enthusiasm is highly visible when people who exercise get together. Walkers and joggers are eager to share their knowledge and experiences. A few tips garnered as the result of such interaction will encourage you to try-out new ideas, techniques, etc. This will help to maintain continuation of your exercise behavior.

Build on Successful Experiences

Emphasize the importance of exercising consistently rather than stressing superior exercise performance. Developing physical fitness and enhancing health take a little time and patience. You should begin to notice some beneficial changes within the first three to four weeks. Focus on these adaptations and use them as a springboard for further gains.

Keep a Progress Chart

It is helpful to keep a daily record because this written information objectively shows the rate and amount of progress that has been achieved. Looking back at the record and observing the gains that have been made can be a source of motivation when one becomes discouraged. The chart should reflect body weight, type, amount, and duration of exercise as well as the resting and exercise heart rates. There should also be room for a short accompanying statement on how you felt during and after the workout (see Figure 2.2).

Weighing oneself prior to and after the workout is important particularly in hot weather when fluid loss can become a major problem. Most of the weight lost during the

DATE	BODY WEIGHT		EXERCISE		INTENSITY**			COMMENTS
	Pre-Exercise	Post-Exercise	Type	Duration*	RHR	THR	PE	

*Time, distance, etc.
**RHR = resting heart rate; THR = training heart rate; PE = perceived exertion

Figure 2.2 Progress chart.

workout is liquid so the difference between pre- and post-exercise weight is an approximation of the amount of fluid loss. This figure should not exceed four to five percent of the body's weight. The loss of one pound of body weight is approximately equal to one pint of fluid loss.[7]

The process of determining and/or approximating fluid loss is one of the functional aspects of the progress chart. Over the long term, a trend for weight loss, distance covered, and heart rates (exercise and resting) will become discernible and you will have a record of improvement.

Exercise to Music

Music provides a sense of rhythm and it tends to take one's mind off the effort associated with walking and jogging. A researcher at Ohio State University tested experienced runners with and without upbeat music.[8] The runners stated that music made the bout of exercise seem easier. They ran both trials, one with and one without music, at the same workload. Measures of working heart rates and blood lactate indicated that the runners were working equally hard on both trials, only their perceptions of the difficulty of the workload were changed. Music can be easily provided indoors and portable radio headsets are very popular among outdoor walkers and joggers.

Set a Definite Time and Place for Exercise

It is best to set a definite time and a convenient place during the initial stages of the exercise program. Resolve to walk or jog at least three times per week and schedule your workout as you would any other important activity. Resist the temptation to replace your workout with some other pursuit that might be more appealing. Skipping workouts becomes habit-forming; the more you do it the easier it becomes. After you become hooked on exercise (it takes three to six months), the time and/or place may be varied to meet changing environmental conditions (weather that is too hot, too humid, too wet, too cold, etc.), work schedules, and other conflicting responsibilities.

When is the best time of day to work out? In the past, I answered by saying that the time of day that fits best into a busy schedule is the best time to exercise. This is still valid but there are other considerations. The best time of day to exercise might be immediately at the end of the work day and before supper. This would serve two purposes: (1) it will metabolize the stress products which have accumulated in the blood during the day, and (2) it will temporarily suppress the appetite resulting in the consumption of fewer calories at supper.

If lack of time is causing you to skip workouts, you might try exercising less frequently but more intensely. While this approach increases the potential for injury, it is better than abandoning the program completely. Exercising less than three times per week will not increase your fitness level but it will lessen the impact of detraining. When you return to your normal exercise routine, your fitness level will not have deteriorated to the point that you will have to start from scratch.

Focus on the Positives

Novice exercisers rather quickly become aware of the negatives associated with working out, such as, muscle soreness, the effort required, sweating, and the feeling of fatigue. But don't let these factors act as deterrents. Concentrate, instead, on your accomplishments. Notice the sense of relaxation after exercise, the increase in energy reserves as you become more physically fit, the loss of body fat and the gain in muscle tissue, the improvement in physical appearance, health status, self concept, and the feeling of general well-being. Focus on the positives and they will keep you motivated and excited about exercise.

Don't Become Obsessive About Exercise

Exercise should consist of activities that are fun and enjoyable but that also allow you to reach your goals. It should be relaxing and recreational, but not obstructive. Don't become so obsessive that you feel and act miserable because you missed a day of exercise. Sometimes unplanned circumstances make it difficult to exercise on a particular day. When that occurs, accept it as one of the two days of rest that will be included in the exercise agenda and pick up the program tomorrow.

If you become ill, do not exercise. Resume activity when your recover. Missing an occasional workout will not detract from the fitness benefits that you have achieved. Later on in this text you will learn about the importance of rest as an integral part of an exercise program.

There Are No Exercise Failures

Physical fitness and health enhancement can be achieved and maintained without competing against others or the time clock. The exercise program that is ultimately adopted should be enjoyable, comfortable, and it should fit your level of physical fitness. Take your time. Walking and/or jogging are not complex skills to perform, and unless you compete in these activities, there are no last place finishes to worry about, no embarrassment with your performance, nor intimidation from others.[9]

Summary

- Only 22% of Americans are active enough to improve their health status.

- The exercise dropout rate is 50% during the initial six months after exercise begins.

- The majority of the "last active" Americans don't exercise because they perceive that they don't have enough time.

- Motivation — a label invented by people to describe a characteristic type of behavior — cannot be measured directly.

- Motivation is any state or condition that causes an organism to produce or inhibit an action or motor response.

- External rewards are effective in the early phase of the exercise program, but it is internal rewards that are most appropriate.

- A moderate level of motivation is optimal — too little is likely to result in failure and too much may result in injury and burnout.

- Most people concede that exercise is good for health enhancement and physical appearance, but the majority of them don't participate.

- Set realistic goals for exercise that are specific and attainable.

▶ Walking is a low impact activity that imposes less demand on the musculo-skeletal system than jogging.

▶ While exercising with a group has a number of advantages, some people prefer to exercise on their own.

▶ Exercise "buddies" can motivate each other and share their knowledge regarding physical fitness.

▶ Spouses, other family members, friends, and co-workers can be important sources of motivation, encouragement, and reinforcement.

▶ Emphasize the importance of exercising consistently rather than stressing superior exercise performance.

▶ REFERENCES

1. Sonstroem, R. J. "Psychological Models," in Dishman, R. K. (Ed.), *Exercise Adherence*, Champaign, IL: Human Kinetics, 1988.

2. Pollock, M. L. "Prescribing Exercise for Fitness and Adherence," in Dishman, R. K. (Ed.), *Exercise Adherence*, Champaign, IL: Human Kinetics, 1988.

3. "Most Less Active Americans Want to be More Active," *NASPE News*, Winter, 1994, p. 11.

4. Dworetzky, J. P., *Psychology*, St. Paul, MN: West Publishing Co., 1998.

5. Knapp, D. N. "Behavioral Management Techniques and Exercise Promotion," in Dishman, R. K. (Ed.), *Exercise Adherence*, Champaign, IL: Human Kinetics, 1988.

6. King, A. C. et. al. "Group- vs Home-Based Exercise Training In Healthy Older Men and Women: A Community Based Clinical Trial," *Journal of the American Medical Association*, 266: 1991, p. 1535.

7. "Are Sports Drinks Better Than Water?" *The Physician and Sportsmedicine*, 20: Feb. 1992, p. 33.

8. Trotter, R. J. "Maybe It's The Music," *Psychology Today*, 8: May, 1984, p. 19.

9. McGlynn, G. *Dynamics of Fitness: A Practical Approach*, Dubuque, IA: William C. Brown, 1987.

3

Guidelines
for
Walking and Jogging

Walking and jogging should become lifelong activities if they are to have a significant and lasting impact on our state of health. A sound program, based upon the guidelines and suggestions presented in this text, has the capacity to improve the quality as well as the quantity of one's life. The health benefits of walking and jogging will be discussed in Chapters 5 and 6, but for now, focus on starting your program correctly. This will ensure the probability of success and thereby promote exercise adherence.

STARTING OUT RIGHT

To be effective, walking, jogging, or any other form of exercise must be performed on a regular basis. Regular participation for two to three months will yield substantial physiological, and psychological benefits that may ultimately provide the motivation to continue. The major problem for the beginning exerciser is to sustain physical activity during the early weeks of participation without losing interest or becoming injured. Enthusiastic beginners, anxious to achieve their goals rapidly tend to overdo it in the early phase of their fitness program. Beginners are faced with a "catch 22" situation: they need enough motivation and enthusiasm to start and maintain the exercise habit, but too much enthusiasm may stimulate them to exercise beyond their capacity. Exercising beyond one's fitness level is not enjoyable, it is extremely uncomfortable, and it is potentially dangerous. If the exerciser attempts to push the program in this manner, negative feelings toward exercise will quickly develop and soon the program with all of its good intentions will be discarded. After all, how many of us are masochistic enough to endure pain and discomfort every exercise session? Consistent participation occurs largely due to our enjoyment of exercise. For normal people, pain and enjoyment are contradictory sensations. Don't become overly impatient for rapid gains — these will come soon enough.

THE MEDICAL EXAM

A medical examination prior to beginning an exercise program is desirable for men 40 years of age or older and for women 50 years of age or older.[1] People who are apparently healthy may participate in low-to-moderate intensity exercises without medical clearance. People who are at higher risk, that is, those who have two or more major coronary risk factors or symptoms suggestive of metabolic disease (diabetes, kidney or liver disease, etc.) should have a medical exam which includes a physician monitored exercise tolerance test. Young adults (college age) can usually start exercising without medical clearance but they should begin within their capacity and progress gradually.

ACHIEVING OBJECTIVES

The exerciser's aims and objectives should help determine the direction of the program and the type of physical activity selected. Weight loss, road race competition, and the development of strength are objectives that suggest different types of physical activities as well as different exercise emphases. The objective of properly conceived exercise programs should be reflected by the manner in which the principles of exercise are manipulated. The degree to which each is emphasized or de-emphasized is the key to accomplishing specific objectives.

TRAINING PRINCIPLES

Each bout of exercise should be preceded by an 8 to 10 minute warm-up and followed by a cool-down period of equal time. Both are integral and important components of a fitness program. Proper warm-up and cool-down procedures contribute to performance and the health and safety of the exerciser. Between these two components is the actual exercise program — in this text walking and jogging — which is based on the following principles of exercise: intensity, frequency, duration, overload, progression, and specificity.

Warming-Up for Exercise

The warm-up is designed to gradually prepare the body for more vigorous exercise. In approximately 10 minutes of warming up, the muscles to be involved in the activity are stretched and heated, and the heart rate is allowed to increase slowly toward that expected during the actual workout. Stretching exercises, rhythmic calisthenics, walking, and slow jogging can be used during the warm-up to prepare the individual for exercise of greater intensity. These activities smooth the transition from inactivity to activity with minimum oxygen deprivation to the heart, muscles, and organs. Without a proper warm-up, the heart rate would escalate rapidly forcing the body to rely upon short-term supplies of fuel to generate the energy for exercise. Circulation does not increase proportionately to heart rate causing a brief interval of time (about two minutes) when the heart and other muscles are not fully supplied with oxygen. This is a potentially dangerous time particularly for those whose circulation is somewhat compromised by heart and blood vessel disease. Though ill advised, the healthy, well-conditioned heart can endure such treatment, but there is some risk.

An example of the healthy heart's response to exercise with and without warming up was illustrated in a study using 44 healthy male subjects ages 21 to 52.[2] All of the subjects had normal electrocardiographic (ECG) responses to running on a treadmill when they were allowed a warm-up of two minutes of easy jogging, but 70% of the same group developed abnormal ECG responses to the same exercise when it was not preceded by a warm-up.

Stretching the muscles occurs when the cardiorespiratory warm-up phase is complete. At this point the walker or jogger should be sweating indicating that the core temperature may be slightly elevated while muscle temperature is substantially elevated.[3] Both responses enhance performance and reduce the risk of physical injury. Muscles are stretched more effectively when heated.

Static stretching is the preferred method for enhancing and maintaining flexibility of the joints and elasticity of muscles and connective tissue. Static stretching consists of slow controlled movements and desired end positions that are held for 15 to 30 seconds. The desired end position should produce a feeling of mild discomfort, but not pain. If pain occurs, you are stretching too forcefully and are in danger of exceeding the elastic properties of muscles. Static stretching is effective for the following reasons: (1) it is not likely to cause injury, (2) it

produces no muscle soreness, (3) it helps to alleviate muscle soreness, and (4) it requires little energy. Static stretches are effective and convenient, they do not require the assistance of a partner, nor is any equipment necessary. Typical stretches for walking and jogging are illustrated in Figures 3.1 through 3.8.

Dynamic or ballistic stretching is not recommended because it forces muscles to pull against themselves. This type of stretching employs bouncing and bobbing movements that activate the stretch reflex (myotatic reflex). Each rapid stretch sends a volley of signals from the stretch reflex to the central nervous system which responds by ordering the stretching muscles to contract instead. If you have dozed off while setting in a chair, you have probably experienced the results of the stretch reflex responding to rapid stretch. Your head drops forward as you nod off causing the neck muscles to stretch rapidly. This sudden dynamic stretch sets the reflexive process in motion that results in rapid contraction of the neck muscles and a quick return of the head to the upright position. The rapid movements in opposite directions can result in muscle soreness and possible injury.

Intensity

Intensity refers to the amount of energy expended per bout of exercise. For the development of physical fitness the American College of Sports Medicine (ACSM) recommends an exercise intensity of 60% to 90% of maximum heart rate.[4] The majority of adults typically exercise at the low end of the range while cardiac patients and normal people with low functional capacity may exercise below the suggested range.[5] The new ACSM guidelines for health enhancement don't mention intensity because it is not important for health enhancement.[6]

WARM-UP STRETCHES

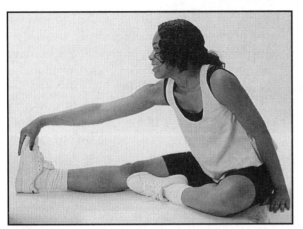

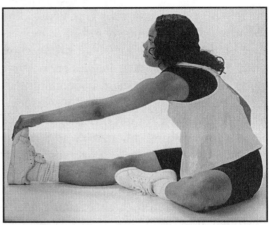

Figure 3.1 Modified Hurdler's Stretch. Sit with the right leg fully extended with the sole of the left foot against the inner right thigh. Keeping the right leg straight, lean forward as far as you can and attempt to reach your foot with the extended right arm. Hold 15 to 30 seconds and switch legs and arms. Stretches the hamstring muscle group in the backs of the thighs.

Figure 3.2 Modified Hurdler's Stretch. Similar to Figure 3.1 but slightly more challenging in that you reach forward with the opposite hand. This will place some stretch on the lower back. Hold 15 to 30 seconds and switch legs and arms.

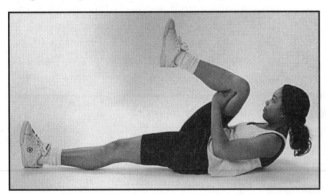

Figure 3.3 Back Stretcher. Lie on your back with hands clasped at the back of the thigh of your right leg. Pull your leg to your chest and hold for 15 to 30 seconds and switch legs. Stretches the lower back.

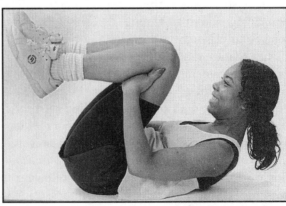

Figure 3.4 Back Stretcher. From the same position as Figure 3.3, clasp your hands behind both thighs and pull both legs to your chest and hold for 15 to 30 seconds. Stretches the lower back.

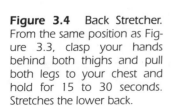

WARM-UP STRETCHES

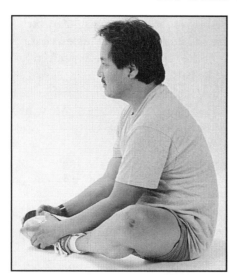

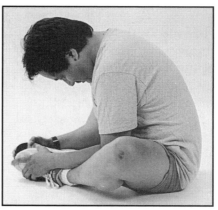

Figure 3.6 Stretching the Inner Thighs and Hips. This is a variation of the exercise in Figure 3.5 but in this case lean forward as you push the knees to the floor. Hold 15 to 30 seconds.

Figure 3.5 Stretching the Inner Thighs and Hips. Seated, bend your knees so that the soles of the feet come together. Use your forearms to push your knees toward the floor. Hold 15 to 30 seconds.

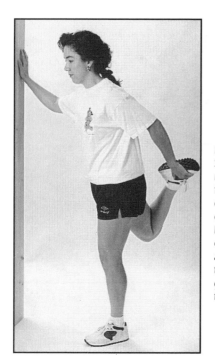

Figure 3.7 Thigh Stretcher. Bend your right leg and pull that foot upward with the opposite hand to avoid excessive bend at the knee. Hold 15 to 30 seconds and switch legs and hands. Stretches the quadriceps muscle group at the front of the thighs.

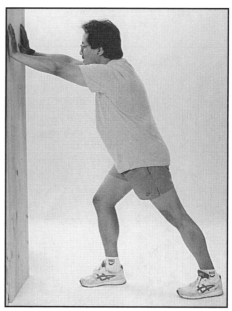

Figure 3.8 Achilles Tendon Stretch. Assume a stride position with the forward leg bent at the knee. The rear leg is straight with the heel planted firmly on the floor. Lean forward until the stretch is felt in the calf and achilles tendon above the heel. Hold 15 to 30 seconds and switch legs. Be sure to point your feet straight ahead.

There are several methods for determining the proper intensity for exercise. One of the most practical is the "talk test." If you cannot carry on a conversation fairly comfortably while walking or jogging, you may be performing at a pace that is too intense for your level of fitness.

A second method involves your perception of the effort. Perceived exertion is an excellent method for monitoring exercise because it includes factors other than heart rate that are indicators of effort. For example it includes overall exertional discomfort and fatigue, rate and depth of breathing, muscle fatigue, and body temperature. These are the subjective impressions of the effort that encompasses sensory input from all of the systems associated with the generation of energy for movement.

The Borg Rate of Perceived Exertion (RPE) and the revised Category — Ratio RPE Scale appears in Figure 3.9. When each value of the original scale on the left in Figure 3.9 is multiplied by 10, it represents a heart rate that is expected to coincide with the descriptor. For example, if the bout of work is perceived by the exerciser to be somewhat hard, it takes a value of 13 which multiplied by 10 yields a heart rate of 130 beats per minute (bpm). Most people exercise between RPEs of 11 to 16 which is fairly light to hard. Heart rates in this range typically equal 130 bpm at the low end of the scale and 160 bpm at the high end. The original scale is the one that is most often used.

A third method for monitoring exercise is by exercise heart rate. There are two ways to determine the exercise heart rate. The first uses a percentage of the maximum heart rate and the second uses a percentage of the cardiac reserve. The estimated maximum heart rate (HR max) must be determined as a first step

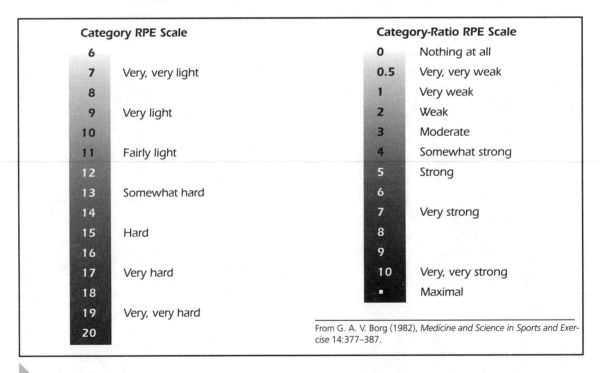

Category RPE Scale		Category-Ratio RPE Scale	
6		0	Nothing at all
7	Very, very light	0.5	Very, very weak
8		1	Very weak
9	Very light	2	Weak
10		3	Moderate
11	Fairly light	4	Somewhat strong
12		5	Strong
13	Somewhat hard	6	
14		7	Very strong
15	Hard	8	
16		9	
17	Very hard	10	Very, very strong
18		∎	Maximal
19	Very, very hard		
20			

From G. A. V. Borg (1982), *Medicine and Science in Sports and Exercise* 14:377–387.

Figure 3.9 RPE scales — original scale on the left; revised scale on the right.

for each method. This is accomplished by subtracting your age in years from the constant 220 so that the HR max for a 20 year old would be:

220 (Constant)
−20 (Age)
―――――――――
200 bpm (HR max)

The HR max decreases with age so that the value for a 50 year old would be 170 bpm (220-50 = 170 bpm). Regardless of age, this method is only an estimate of the HR max. The HR that the exerciser will attempt to maintain during exercise is referred to as the target HR.

The first method for establishing the target HR uses a percentage of the HR max. The ACSM recommends that people exercise at an intensity level somewhere between the range of 60% to 90% of the HR max. A person in average physical condition would select the middle of the range or 70% to 80% of the HR max. Our 20 year old with a HR max of 200 bpm would have a target HR of 140 bpm to 160 bpm. This is computed as follows:

200 bpm (HR max)	200 bpm (HR max)
× .7	× .8
140 bpm	160 bpm

People who are in better physical condition would select a higher percentage of their HR max while those in poorer condition would select a lower percentage.

A more sophisticated approach for determining the target HR is by the Karvonen Method. This method employs the exerciser's resting HR, which is a crude measure of physical fitness, and the cardiac reserve which is the difference between the HR max and the resting HR. Fit people generally have lower resting HRs and higher cardiac reserves than unfit people. The target for a 20 year old who is in average physical condition with a resting HR

of 70 bpm is calculated in the following manner by the Karvonen Method:

1. Calculate HR max as before

220
−20
―――――――――
200 bpm (HR max)

2. The Karvonen Formula is:

THR = Cardiac reserve × T1% + RHR

Where:

THR = target heart rate
Cardiac reserve = HR max − RHR
T1% = training intensity
        (Get this value from Table 3.1)
RHR = resting heart rate

Therefore:

THR = (HR max − RHR) × T1% + RHR
     = (200 − 70) × .70 + 70
     = 161 bpm

The resting HR must be known in order to use the Karvonen Method. Since many factors affect the RHR, it is best to establish this value under standard conditions. Take the pulse rate (HR) while sitting on the side of the bed after awakening in the morning. Take the pulse rate after sitting for about two minutes. Repeat the procedure for 4 to 5 consecutive days and average all of the pulse rates. This should produce a good representation of the normal resting heart rate.

 Table 3.1   *Guidelines for Selecting Training Intensity Level*

Fitness Level	Intensity Level (%)
Low	60
Fair	65
Average	70
Good	75
Excellent	80 – 90

Learning to take HR by palpating the pulse is a skill that must be developed. The two most practical sites and the ones most often used are the radial and carotid arteries. See Figures 3.10 and 3.11. The radial pulse is palpated at the thumb side of the wrist with the hand held palm up. The carotid pulse is felt in the large arteries at either side of the neck. Use the first two fingers of either hand to count the pulse rate in either location.

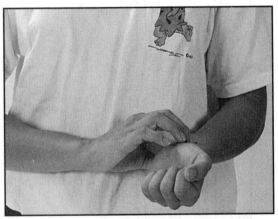

Figure 3.10   Taking the radial pulse at the wrist with the fingers.

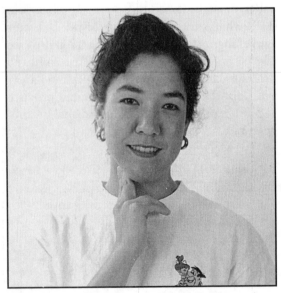

Figure 3.11   Taking the carotid pulse at the neck.

Care should be taken when palpating the carotid pulse because the arteries in the neck are sensitive to pressure. Excessive pressure stretches the arteries and stimulates specialized receptors therein that respond reflexively by slowing the heart's rate of beating. This leads to an underestimation of the actual heart rate. To circumvent this effect, the pressure applied to the carotid should not exceed the amount required to feel the pulse.

Frequency

The ACSM recommends that physical activity be performed 3 to 5 days per week. Less than 3 days per week is not enough of a stimulus to improve fitness and more than 5 days per week results in diminishing returns, staleness, and increases the likelihood of injury.[7] The intensity and duration of exercise should help with the selection of its frequency. For example, low intensity exercise of moderate duration (20 to 40 minutes), such as strolling (walking at 3 mph) could be performed everyday without resulting in orthopedic problems or staleness.

Exercise does not have to be performed in one continuous bout to be beneficial. It can be split into several shorter sessions during the day. Two groups of male subjects exercised for a total of 30 minutes a day, three times per week, at 65% to 75% of their HR max.[8] One of the groups exercised continuously for 30 minutes while the other group split the 30 minutes into three 10 minute exercise sessions. At the end of eight weeks, the fitness level of both groups improved but the one-exercise session group improved more. However, both groups lost the same amount of weight during the course of the study. Short bouts of exercise spaced throughout the day is a realistic exercise option for very busy people.

Days of rest are an important component of any training program. These are needed for physical and mental recuperation. Exercisers who don't take days off run the risk of burning out or becoming stale. There is a fine line between the amount of exercise that produces maximum gains and the amount of exercise that results in the negative effects (staleness) associated with overtraining. Overtraining occurs when exercisers do too much too often. The signs of this phenomenon are:

1. A feeling of chronic fatigue and listlessness.
2. Inability to make further fitness gains (or there may be a loss of fitness).
3. A sudden loss of weight.
4. An increase of five beats or more in the resting heart rate, taken in the morning prior to getting out of bed.
5. Loss of enthusiasm for working out (the exerciser no longer looks forward to the workout).
6. Vulnerability to injury and illness.
7. Feelings of anger.
8. Depression.

Staleness may be both psychological (lack of variety in the program or boredom after years of training) and physiological. It is probably a combination of both, but the treatment is the same: either stop training for a few days to a few weeks (depends upon the severity of staleness) or cut back substantially. In either case, rebuild and regain fitness gradually. Prevention is the best treatment. Recognize the signs and adjust accordingly before staleness becomes a problem.

Duration

Duration refers to the length of each bout of exercise. In its latest guidelines, the ACSM recommended that exercise should last a minimum of 30 minutes and be performed most days of the week. This amount of exercise will improve the health status and fitness level of sedentary people. But this should be considered a minimum program. Epidemiological data have shown that expending 1000 kcals to 2000 kcals per week — the equivalent of walking or jogging 10 to 20 miles per week — resulted in fewer heart attacks and longer life.[9]

Overload and Progression

Overload involves subjecting the various systems of the body (muscular, cardiorespiratory, skeletal, etc) to greater physical demand. Progression represents the manner and the time when these demands are applied. The application of periodic overload forces the body to adapt, and in the process, physical fitness is developed. Exercisers must overload on a schedule of systematic progression for improvement to occur. But, when the desired level of fitness has been attained the exerciser switches from the development of fitness to the maintenance of fitness. At this point, the practices of overload and progression are no longer needed.

For walking and jogging, overload can be applied systematically and progressively. This can be accomplished by one or a combination of the following: (1) gradually increase the distance, (2) decrease the time that it takes to cover a specified distance, and (3) participate more frequently. A good rule of thumb is to increase the frequency and duration of exercise while holding intensity steady. Intensity can be increased after a base of fitness has been developed.

Three observations might be noted regarding the application of overload: (1) be patient so as not to exercise beyond your capacity,

(2) improvements in fitness are greatest during the first three months of training and continue to occur for a period of time but in smaller increments, and (3) overload should be applied only when individuals are ready to accept a new challenge.

Specificity

The body adapts according to the specific type of stress to which it is subjected. The muscles, systems, and organs used in any given activity are the ones that adapt and they do so in the specific way in which they are used. Jogging does not prepare one for swimming and swimming does not prepare one for cycling because these activities are sufficiently different from each other. The legs are stressed by jogging in a manner that is unique to that activity. The adaptations that result from jogging provide little carryover to the leg kick for swimming.

Competitors who are attempting to maximize their physical performance in a given activity are locked into a training program that is task-specific. This involves repetitive overloading of the muscles that are used in the event. Triathalon training is a good example of the practical use of the principle of specificity. Triathletes must train vigorously in all three events of the triathalon because no combination of training for any two of them will result in substantial improvement in the third.

People who walk and/or jog for health and fitness are not confined solely to these activities. They can occasionally swim, cycle, play tennis, racquetball or other games for fun and variety. Walking and jogging are the core of the fitness program but participants have the option of engaging in other activities on occasion should they desire. At least two days of

weight training are a must. Weight training should supplement walking and jogging because it stresses the total muscular system in ways that cannot be achieved by walking and jogging. Many people who exercise for health reasons enjoy participating in more than one physical activity. This is called cross-training. Still others prefer one activity because they enjoy it and it meets their needs. The point is to select an activity or activities that provide enjoyment and fulfill your health and fitness needs. Walking and jogging qualify for both.

Cooling Down After Exercise

Cooling down after exercise is as important as warming up. Just as the body was allowed to speed up gradually, it must also be allowed to slow down gradually. The body is not analogous to an auto engine that can be turned on and off with the twist of a key. Cool-down should last about 8 to 10 minutes. The first phase of cooling down should consist of walking or some other light activity and the second phase should consist of the same stretching exercises that were performed during the warm-up.

Phase One: Light Activity

Five minutes of continuous light activity causes rhythmical muscle contractions that prevent the pooling of blood and helps to move blood back to the heart for redistribution to the vital organs. This boost to circulation after exercise is an essential component of the cool-down period. Inactivity during this time forces the heart to compensate for the reduced volume of blood returning to it by maintaining a high pumping rate. The exerciser runs the risk of dizziness, fainting, and perhaps more serious consequences associated with diminished blood flow. The most serious of these consequences is sudden death. The recovery period following exercise represents a potential hazard if it is not approached properly. While sudden death during or immediately after exercise is a rare event, it does occur, and the recovery period is one of the most likely times.

The worst possible cool-down procedure after fast walking or jogging is to stop all activity and stand still. The blood vessels in the legs that were dilated during exercise remain that way for a time after exercise so that blood pools in the leg veins. The downward force of gravity is an impediment to the return of blood from the legs to the heart. Blood vessel dilation plus the force of gravity reduces blood flow to the heart which limits the amount available for the body's various systems. Because venous return of blood to the heart is reduced, the systolic blood pressure drops but heart rate remains high. The systolic pressure represents the pressure of the blood against the artery walls when the heart contracts. While the pressure is dropping, the hormone norepinephrine rises in the blood stream. Norepinephrine constricts blood vessels and will, under normal circumstances, raise the blood pressure. Many authorities contend that the rise in norepinephrine after exercise is a safety mechanism in which the body reflexively attempts to maintain a proper blood pressure. However, the stand-still posture after exercise overcomes the action of norepinephrine so that the pressure drops anyway. The rise in norepinephrine, the drop in blood pressure along with a relatively high heart rate represents circulation that is out of kilter. This set of events may be the triggering mechanism for the onset of irregular heart beats that can lead to sudden death.

The key to avoiding or at least substantially reducing the probability of sudden death after exercise is to keep moving. Walking at a moderate speed for five minutes will prevent the pooling of blood in the legs because the contracting muscles squeeze the veins sending more blood back to the heart. The rhythmic contractions of the leg muscles, referred to as the "muscle pump," act as a second heart significantly assisting it to meet the body's elevated circulatory demand. Another plus for light physical activity during cool-down is that it hastens the removal of lactic acid that accumulates in the muscles.

It is imperative to continue to walk if you become nauseated after exercise. If you feel dizzy to the point that walking is not possible nor advisable, it is best to lie down on your back. This position prevents the pooling of blood in the legs because the horizontal position nullifies the force of gravity. The feeling of nausea and the subsequent vomiting that might occur when people exercise beyond their capacity is another of the body's safety mechanisms. Vomiting kicks the blood pressure up toward normal and within minutes, the exerciser begins to feel better.

Phase Two: Stretching Exercises

The second phase of cool-down should focus upon the same stretching exercises that were used during the warm-up period. You will probably note that stretching is tolerated more comfortably after exercise due to the increase in muscle temperature. Stretching at this time helps prevent muscle soreness. Bent leg sit-ups should be added to the routine. Strong abdominal muscles are a postural aid because they provide support for the upper torso. Modified sit-ups should be done by those who cannot do sit-ups correctly due to unused and weak abdominals. Correct performance requires that the back be rounded as the participant sits up. See Figures 3.12 through 3.15.

COOL-DOWN EXERCISES

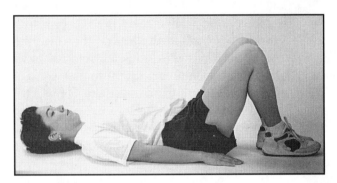

Figure 3.12 Modified Sit-Up (Part 1). Lie on your back with knees bent and heels close to the buttocks. Arms are extended at your sides.

Figure 3.13 Modified Sit-Up (Part 2). Curl up with straight arms until your fingertips contact your knees and return to the starting position. This is a lead up to more strenuous abdominal exercises. Start with 10 repetitions and progress from there.

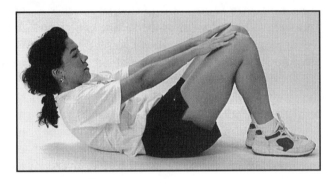

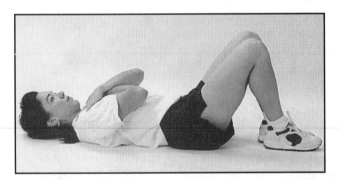

Figure 3.14 Sit-Up (Part 1). Lie on your back, knees bent, feet close to buttocks, arms folded across the chest.

Figure 3.15 Sit-Up (Part 2). Curl up until your shoulder blades lose contact with the floor and return to the starting position (Part 1). Start with 10 repetitions and progress from there.

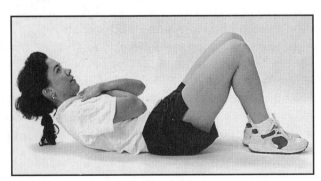

WALKING FOR HEALTH AND FITNESS

Walking is the natural form of locomotion for human beings. All humans walk unless some form of disability prevents it. For those who are sedentary, walking is a safe, easy, economical, and convenient way to start exercising. It can be a lead-up activity for more strenuous exercise or its intensity can be manipulated so that it can be the primary or sole method of exercise. A well-conceived walking program that includes the appropriate pacing, frequency, duration, and performance techniques can meet health, fitness, and racing objectives. This text focuses on health and fitness walking and will not cover race walking. Race walking involves a unique style of locomotion that requires instruction, knowledge, skill, and practice to perfect. This is beyond the scope of this text. Health and fitness walking rather than competitive walking require few special skills and yet are effective in producing fitness and health enhancement.

These Shoes Were Made for Walking

Walking is a low impact activity that can be performed indoors or outdoors, in different climate conditions, and on varying types of terrain. Shoes designed specifically for exercise walking for different terrains have been developed and are one of the essential components for this activity. Appropriate footwear adds to the enjoyment of walking and reduces the likelihood of incurring a walking-related injury.

The following guidelines should help in the selection of proper walking shoes:

1. The shoes should be well padded at the heel to absorb the impact of landing. (See Figure 3.16) It is imperative that women's shoes be well padded in this area because they tend to land with more force per body weight than men at all walking speeds. The heels on all walking shoes should be 1/2 to 3/4 of an inch higher than the sole.

2. The shoes should fit snugly at the heel and instep (the arched upper part of the foot) and it should follow the foot's natural conformation.

3. The outer sole should be constructed of durable solid rubber or carbon rubber for long wear. The tread should be designed for good traction.

4. The inner soles of good walking shoes should include removable arch supports and heel cups. These can be removed after a workout so that they can air out and dry.

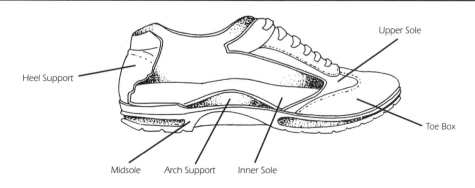

Figure 3.16   A typical walking shoe.

5. The upper portion of walking shoes should be constructed from leather, synthetic fabrics, or a combination of both. These materials enhance breathability and foot comfort.

6. All walking shoes are relatively lightweight. Unless you are a competitor, it is not necessary nor advisable to purchase the lightest shoes on the market. Foot protection rather than shoe weight is most important for those who walk for health and fitness.

7. Shoes should be selected for function rather than color or fashion.

8. Beginners might do well to purchase their first couple of pairs of walking shoes from a sporting goods store that specializes in sports footwear. Their professional sales people can assist in the selection and proper sizing of the shoes.

The Energy Cost of Walking

Walkers never lose contact with the surface upon which they are traversing. A walker's advancing or striding foot lands before the rear foot leaves the ground. The rear foot supports the weight of the body while the advancing foot is swinging forward. Also there is a brief period when both feet are simultaneously in contact with the ground. At slow speeds, the normal walking gait, with its relaxed arm swing, is a very efficient form of locomotion which actually conserves and reduces energy expenditure. To some extent, this is a drawback to the development of physical fitness. But research indicates that walking efficiency decreases and energy expenditure increases as walking speed increases. The faster you walk, the more calories you burn. This is not the case with jogging where speed is irrelevant. Jogging a 10 minute mile is much more comfortable yet burns about the same number of calories as jogging a six minute mile. Table 3.2 provides a comparison of the caloric expenditure for walking at different speeds for selected body weights. This table presents walking speed in miles per hour (mph) and each speed is translated into minutes and seconds to walk one mile at that pace. For example, walking at 3.5 mph, the walker would cover the mile distance in 17 minutes and 10 seconds (17:10). If the walker weighed 150 lbs, he or she would expend 4.2 Kcals/min. or 72 Kcals per mile (17.17 × 4.2 = 72). Note that seconds must be converted into hundredths of a minute by dividing the number of seconds by 60 (10/60 = .166). Kcals (kilocalories) is the symbol used to denote the caloric value of foods and this symbol will be used throughout the text.

Table 3.2 indicates that the Kcal cost of walking increases significantly at speeds above 3.5 mph. This is primarily due to the fact that we become less efficient as speed increases above 3.5 mph. The differences in Kcals expended in walking 5 mph versus 3 mph is 34 Kcals per mile for a 150 lb person. If these speeds are maintained for an hour the difference is 318 Kcals.

Body weight also has an impact on energy expenditure for both walking and jogging. Walking at 3.5 mph, a 120 lb person burns 3.4 Kcals/minute while a 210 lb person burns 5.9 Kcals/minute. This is a difference of 2.5 Kcals/min for every minute walked and a 150 Kcal difference for 60 minutes.

The energy expenditure of walking can be increased by vigorously swinging the arms, by swinging hand-held weights, by walking up hills, or any combination of these techniques. A word of caution: vigorously swinging hand-held weights can result in shoulder soreness or injury. It might also lead to an abnormally high blood pressure response if the weights are gripped tightly. It is safer to vigorously swing the arms without weights — the difference in

Table 3.2 The Energy Cost of Walking in Kcals/Minute

Body Weight (lbs.)	Walking Speed (mph)						
	2.0 (30 m/m)*	2.5 (24 m/m)	3.0 (20 m/m)	3.5 (17:10 m/m)	4.0 (15 m/m)	4.5 (13:20 m/m)	5.0 (12 m/m)
120	2.3	2.6	3.0	3.4	4.4	5.6	7.2
150	2.8	3.3	3.7	4.2	5.6	7.0	9.0
180	3.4	4.0	4.5	5.0	6.7	84	10.8
210	4.0	4.6	5.2	5.9	7.8	9.9	12.6

*m/m = minutes per mile

Note: To find the Kcals expended per minute locate the appropriate body weight and move horizontally to the right until you reach your speed of walking. The kcals expended per minute is located where the two intersect. For example, a 180 lb. person walking at 4 mph would expend 6.7 kcals/min. Kcals per mile would equal 100.5. (15 m/m × 6.7 = 100.5 kcals/m). If this same individual walked at 4 mph for 40 minutes the Kcals expended would be 40 × 6.7 = 268 kcals.

caloric expenditure and fitness development will not be significant. Do not wear ankle weights because these may distort the natural gait and lead to injury. Hill walking significantly increases energy demand and should be a part of the program. Approach hill walking cautiously at first, attempt steeper and longer hills as fitness improves, and walk the hills faster (See Table 3.3).

The Mechanics of Walking

Walking at 3 mph is considered to be casual walking or strolling; at 4 mph walking progresses to brisk or fitness walking; and 5 mph or faster walking becomes race pace. The faster one walks, the faster the arms swing. In fact the converse is true — walking speed may be increased by concentrating on rapidly swinging

Table 3.3 Calories Used Walking Uphill*

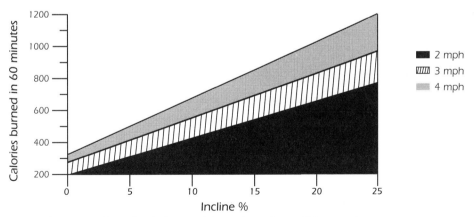

Approximate number of calories used in an hour by a 150 pound person walking uphill at different speeds on various inclines. Most hilly streets have inclines of 10 to 25%.

the arms because leg speed tends to follow arm speed. Obviously, walking at 3 mph does not require a rapid arm turnover but walking at 5 mph does. However, my purpose is not to produce race walkers but rather to provide solid information to encourage regular participation in health and fitness walking. Rapid speeds are not necessary for health enhancement nor for the development of fitness. But vigorous arm swinging is just as important for increasing the energy requirements of walking as it is for increasing speed. Walking at a brisk 4 mph with energetic arm swinging materially increases the energy cost of walking.

Proper walking technique requires an erect, but not stiff posture. (See Figure 3.17) Do not look down at the walking surface by bending your neck (see Figure 3.18). Instead, hold your head erect and scan the road surface with your eyes only. If you bend your neck forward to watch where you are stepping, you will be leaning forward. This position puts a strain on

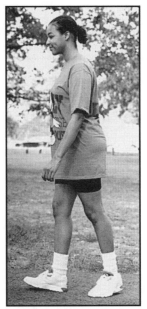

Figure 3.18 Incorrect Walking Posture. Head and neck forward, eyes looking down.

the lower back, upper back, and neck. It requires the static contraction of extraneous muscles and is wasteful of energy.

The arms should be held with a 90° bend at the elbows. The hands should be loosely closed and relaxed. (See Figure 3.19) For efficiency, the arms should be swung vertically and the hands should travel no higher than the ear lobes. The arms are bent at 90 degrees throughout the entirety of the swing. You will find it very difficult to increase walking speed if you swing your arms from the shoulders in pendulum style. (See Figure 3.20)

In walking, the initial point of contact with the ground is the heel of the foot. This applies to all styles of walking from casual strolling to race walking. Foot placement changes as speed increases. During normal gait walking or strolling, the feet land on either side of an imaginary line that proceeds in the direction of travel. See Figure 3.21. As speed increases to brisk walking, the stride lengthens and the feet land closer to the imaginary line. In race walking, the feet would actually land on the line.

The knee should be slightly bent when the heel contacts the ground. The landing foot rolls forward accepting the weight of the body as the rear foot provides a forceful push from the toes (see Figure 3.22). This is repeated rhythmically with every step.

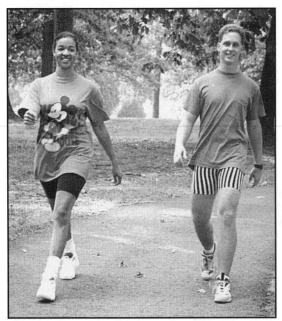

Figure 3.17 Proper Walking Posture. Erect but relaxed.

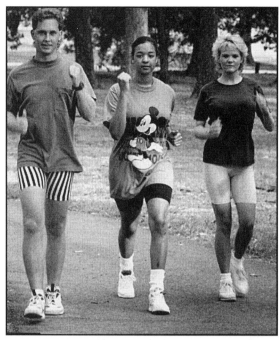

Figure 3.19 *Speed Walking or Fitness Walking.* The arms are bent 90 degrees at the elbows and swung vigorously. The hands should not go higher than the ear lobes on the upswing.

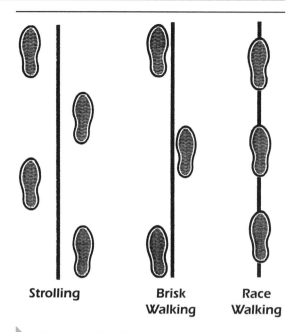

Strolling   **Brisk Walking**   **Race Walking**

Figure 3.21 Changes in foot placement for various walking speeds.

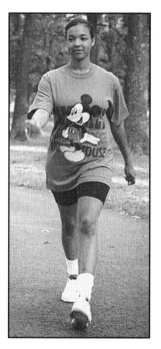

Figure 3.20 Normal-Gaited Walking. Arms swinging pendulum-style.

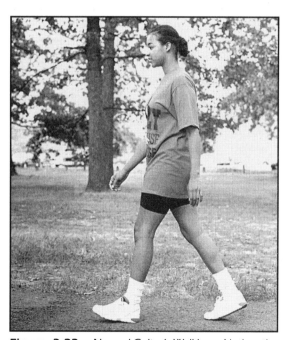

Figure 3.22 Normal-Gaited Walking. Notice the heel strike on landing, the knee bent on receipt of the body weight, and the push-off from the toes of the rear foot.

Walking Tips — A Summary

1. Beginners should walk at a comfortable pace.

2. Posture is erect, but not stiff.

3. Arms should be bent at a 90 degree angle at the elbows.

4. Hands should be loosely clenched.

5. Arm swing should be vigorous with the hands traveling no higher than the ear lobes. This will increase the caloric expenditure of walking by 5% to 10%.

6. The striding leg lands on the heel and the force rolls up to the toes.

7. The rear foot provides a strong push-off.

8. The arms and legs move contralaterally, that is, the right arm and left leg move forward together and the left arm and right leg move forward together.

9. The effort can be increased safely by lengthening the distance, increasing the speed, swinging the arms vigorously, and walking up hills.

10. Walk on alternate days and gradually increase the distance. When you can walk for 30 to 45 minutes without undue fatigue, you can increase the frequency to 4 to 5 days per week. If it meets your objectives, intensity can be increased after frequency and duration have been satisfied.

▶ JOGGING FOR HEALTH AND FITNESS

Jogging is the activity of choice for millions of Americans. Both fitness and health objectives can be attained expeditiously with a jogging program and, of course, this is part of its appeal. A short list of the benefits that accrue from jogging follow:

▶ It is one of the best activities for conditioning the cardiorespiratory system as well as most of the body's largest and most powerful muscles.

▶ It is excellent for weight loss and weight maintenance.

▶ It is an excellent relaxer and stress reducer.

▶ It has a beneficial effect on the risk factors for cardiovascular disease.

▶ It reduces susceptibility to many other chronic diseases.

▶ It can be performed recreationally, competitively, alone, or with others.

These Shoes Were Made for Jogging

The most important investment that a prospective jogger can make is the purchase of quality shoes. Care should be exercised in their selection because an appropriate, well fitting pair of shoes may prevent or alleviate blisters, shin splints, ankle, knee, and hip joint injuries.

Shoes made especially for jogging have some common characteristics (see Figure 3.23). The heel should be about one-half inch higher than the sole and it should be well padded. The sole should consist of two separate layers with the outer layer made of a durable rubberized compound for traction and longevity. The inner layer should be thick and pliable and made of shock absorbing material. It is desirable for the heel and sole to flare out so the impact with the ground can be distributed over a wide area. This is critical because the jogger's foot hits the ground 600-750 times per mile with each foot strike absorbing a force equivalent to three times the body weight. It should come as no surprise that the incidence of stress injuries rises linearly with the number of miles jogged.

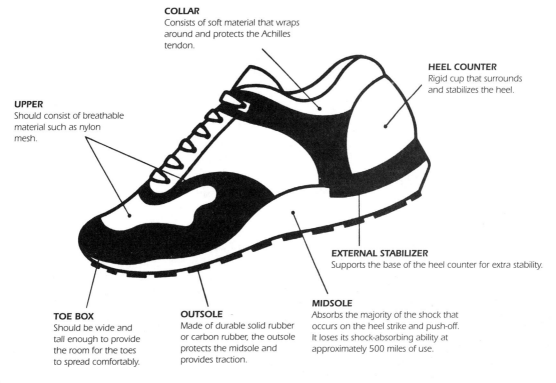

COLLAR
Consists of soft material that wraps around and protects the Achilles tendon.

HEEL COUNTER
Rigid cup that surrounds and stabilizes the heel.

UPPER
Should consist of breathable material such as nylon mesh.

EXTERNAL STABILIZER
Supports the base of the heel counter for extra stability.

TOE BOX
Should be wide and tall enough to provide the room for the toes to spread comfortably.

OUTSOLE
Made of durable solid rubber or carbon rubber, the outsole protects the midsole and provides traction.

MIDSOLE
Absorbs the majority of the shock that occurs on the heel strike and push-off. It loses its shock-absorbing ability at approximately 500 miles of use.

Figure 3.23 A typical jogging shoe.

Flexibility, another characteristic of a good shoe, can be determined by grasping the heel in one hand and the toe in the other and bending it. If it does not bend easily, it is too stiff and inflexible for jogging.

Proper fit is another important factor. The shoes should be one-half inch longer than the longest toe and the toe box should allow enough room for the toes to spread. The toe box should be high enough not to pinch down the toes. The heel of the foot should fit snugly in the padded heel of the shoe for maximal support and minimal friction. The shoe should have a good, firm arch support.

When purchasing a pair of shoes, one should wear the same type of sock that will be worn when jogging in order to minimize errors in sizing. Some attention should also be given to shoe maintenance. It's best to own more than one pair of shoes so they can be rotated from workout to workout. However, one pair will suffice if they are allowed to dry between workouts.

Shoes should be inspected periodically and discarded if they wear deep into the outer layer. As the shoe wears, the angle of the foot strike changes producing vectors for forces at sites in the legs and hips to which the jogger is unaccustomed. This increases the likelihood of injury and enforced idleness for a period of time.

Thirty percent of the shock absorbing qualities of jogging shoes dissipates at about 500 miles of wear regardless of price, brand, or type of construction.[10] At this point it is best to replace your jogging shoes.

Purchase your jogging shoes from a store that specializes in the sale of sports footwear. Tell them your price range and let the professional sales people suggest shoes in that range that are appropriate to your needs.

The Energy Cost of Jogging

The energy cost of jogging for a particular body weight is about the same regardless of speed. In fact, the *net energy* cost of jogging (the total Kcals used minus the Kcals that would be used while at rest) is exactly the same. The *total or gross Kcals* used (resting Kcals plus net Kcals) varies a bit. Refer to Table 3.4 for the gross and net Kcals used by selected body weights at different speeds. The first line for each weight presents the gross and net Kcals per minute while the second line presents the gross and net Kcals per mile. Note that the net Kcals do not change with speed but there is a slight change in the gross Kcals with changing speeds for the same body weight. An individual weighing 120 lbs uses

the same number of net Kcals per mile whether he or she jogs at 4 mph or 8 mph. At 8 mph, the individual will be generating energy at twice the rate expended at 4 mph but will only be jogging for half the time so that the net Kcals expended per mile will be the same. The gross expenditure per mile actually decreases as speed increases but the reduction is insignificant. Joggers can shorten the workout by running faster and still use the same number of Kcals per mile, or they can jog slower at a more comfortable rate of speed for a longer period of time and expend about the same number of total Kcals.

The net caloric cost of jogging one mile is twice that of walking a mile on level ground at moderate speeds. But at higher rates of walking speed (5 mph or faster), the caloric cost of running one mile is only 10% more than walking one mile (see Table 3.5). Notice that the net energy expenditure for walking is quite stable up to 3.5 mph. Above this speed, the net Kcals increase rapidly so that the energy expenditure for walking and jogging come closer together. A 150 lb. person walking and jogging at the same speed expends similar amounts of energy

Table 3.4 Gross/Net Kcal Expenditure for Jogging*

Body Weight (lbs.)	MPH SPEED MIN PER MILE	4.0 15.0	5.0 12.0	6.0 10.0	7.0 8:30	8.0 7:30	9.0 6:40	10.0 6.0
120	Kcals (min)	6.5/5.5	7.8/6.9	9.2/8.3	10.8/9.8	12/11.1	13.3/12.4	14.8/13.8
	Kcals (mile)	97/83	94/83	92/83	92/83	90/83	89/83	89/83
150	Kcals (min)	8.1/6.9	9.8/8.7	11.5/10.4	13.4/12.2	15.1/13.9	16.8/15.6	18.5/17.3
	Kcals (mile)	121/104	118/104	115/105	114/104	113/104	112/104	111/104
180	Kcals (min)	9.7/8.3	11.8/10.4	13.8/12.5	16.1/14.7	18.1/16.7	20.1/18.7	22.2/20.8
	Kcals (mile)	146/125	141/125	138/125	137/125	136/125	134/125	133/125
210	Kcals (min)	11.3/9.7	13.8/12.2	16.1/14.6	18.8/17.2	21.1/19.5	23.4/21.9	25.8/24.3
	Kcals (mile)	170/146	165/146	161/146	160/146	158/146	156/146	155/146

*The first number in each set is the gross Kcals; the second number is the net Kcals. The first set of numbers for each body weight is the Kcals per minute for each speed; the second set is the Kcals per mile for each speed. Example: A 150 lb person jogging at 6 mph will expend 11.5 gross Kcals/min; 10.4 net Kcals/min; 115 gross Kcals/mile; 105 net Kcals/mile.

Table 3.5   Gross/Net Kcal Expenditure for Walking*

Body Weight (lbs.)	MPH SPEED MIN PER MILE	2.0 30	2.5 24	3.0 20	3.5 17:08	4.0 15	4.5 13:20	5.0 12
120	Kcals (min)	2.3/1.4	2.6/1.8	3.0/2.1	3.3/2.5	4.4/3.5	5.6/4.7	7.2/6.3
	Kcals (mile)	69/42	63/42	59/42	57/42	66/52	75/63	86/75
150	Kcals (min)	2.9/1.7	3.3/2.2	3.7/2.6	4.2/3.0	5.5/4.3	7.0/5.9	9.0/7.8
	Kcals (mile)	87/52	79/52	74/52	72/52	82/65	93/78	108/94
180	Kcals (min)	3.5/2.1	4.0/2.6	4.5/3.2	5.0/3.7	6.6/5.2	8.4/7.1	10.8/9.4
	Kcals (mile)	104/63	95/63	89/63	86/63	99/78	112/94	129/113
210	Kcals (min)	4.0/2.4	4.6/3.0	5.2/3.7	5.8/4.3	7.7/6.1	9.8/8.3	12.6/11.0
	Kcals (mile)	121/173	111/73	104/73	100/73	115/92	131/110	151/132

*The first number in each set is the gross Kcals; the second number is the net Kcals. The first set of numbers for each body weight is the Kcals per minute for each speed; the second set is the Kcals per mile for each speed. Example: A 150 lb person walking at 3.5 mph will expend 4.2 gross Kcals/min; 3.0 net Kcals/min; 72 gross Kcals/mile; 52 net Kcals/mile.

on a per mile basis. For example, if this 150 lb. person walks and jogs at 5 mph, the difference in energy expended per mile is only 10 Kcals. Examine Tables 3.4 and 3.5 closely and compare the two for Kcals burned for different body weights and different speeds. Based upon your exercise objectives, the data in these tables may contribute to the selection of the exercise mode that is right for you.

The Mechanics of Jogging

A comfortable erect posture with head level encourages correct body alignment for jogging (see Figures 3.24 and 3.25). The eyes should survey the road in front of you for obstacles and irregular terrain but the neck should not be bent in the forward position. Do not look directly in front of your feet because this detracts from jogging efficiency and it leads to muscle strain in the neck and lower back if this posture is maintained for any length of time.

The hands, which are loosely closed, should be carried slightly lower than the elbows for energy conservation and comfort. This posture tends to relax the neck and shoulders. The low hand position mitigates against the generation of the powerful pumping action from the arms, but this is not necessary for jogging. Sprinters require power from the arm swing; joggers swing the arms for rhythm and balance. The

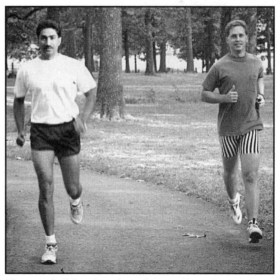

Figure 3.24   Jogging Form. Erect but relaxed posture.

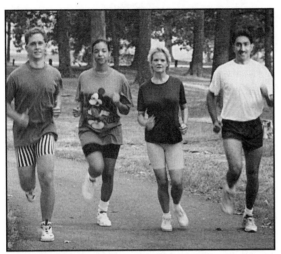

Figure 3.25 Correct Jogging Form. Erect and relaxed. Many people prefer jogging with a group.

arms should be swung backward and forward but should not cross in front of the body.

The jogging stride should be short and compact with the foot landing beneath the knee. This is an aid to keeping the body erect and prevents overstriding. The jogger should land softly on the heel and rock up through the ball of the foot to the toes for the push-off. The body weight transfers from the heel, along the outside edge of the foot to the toes. This distributes the impact over a greater surface area and for a longer period of time and results in smooth energy-efficient locomotion. The landing should be essentially noiseless.

The major difference between walking and jogging is that the body is airborne during each stride while jogging. The airborne or "float phase" accounts for about 30% of the stride length. The airborne phase represents one of the primary reasons that the energy cost of jogging is higher than walking. It takes more energy to propel the body into the air with each stride. Overstriding is to be avoided. When the ankle is forward of the knee upon landing, the foot acts as a brake to forward

motion. This not only reduces the efficiency of jogging but it puts stress upon the knee joint increasing the probability of injury.

The mechanical factors that make jogging such a good aerobic conditioner are the very ones that can produce injury. The fact that joggers are airborne with every step results in a high impact landing. The ground reaction force when the foot strikes the surface coupled with the subsequent push-off that propels the body upward is approximately equal to three times the body weight. Since the average jogger steps between 600 and 750 strides per mile knees, hips, and feet absorb the shock of landing that many times. Multiply these values by the number of miles covered in a week and you can understand the accumulative forces operating on the jogger. But, joggers make a number of biomechanical adjustments that help to dissipate the shock. For example, the flexed position of the knee and ankle when the heel strikes the ground allows the contracting muscles to stabilize the involved joints. In the contracted position, the muscles act as shock absorbers that diffuse the impact of landing. By the time the shock reaches the hip joint it has been effectively reduced to one-sixth of its original intensity. These adjustments allow joggers to run for many years without serious injuries or premature wear of the joints. Despite this remarkable adaptability, most joggers sustain an injury or two sometime during their many years of jogging. Fortunately, most of these are minor and respond well to rest or treatment.

Jogging Tips: A Summary

1. Sedentary people should ease into jogging. Begin by walking and progress to a combination of walking and jogging. In the beginning, spend much more time walking. As fitness improves reduce walking time and

increase jogging time until eventually, you will be able to jog for the entire exercise session.

2. Keep the intensity (pace) at a low level. Increase frequency and duration before increasing intensity.

3. Jogging posture features an erect but not stiff, body position with head level and eyes moving to scan the road ahead.

4. Hands should be slightly lower than the elbows during the arm swing because this promotes relaxation of the neck, shoulders, and jaw.

5. Do not swing your arms across your body because this results in rotational sway that decreases efficiency.

6. Land on the heel so that the large muscles of the legs will absorb the shock of landing.

7. A quality pair of jogging shoes is a must, particularly if you must run on city streets and sidewalks.

8. GOOD LUCK!

Summary

▶ A medical exam is desirable prior to starting an exercise program for men 40 years of age or older and for women 50 years of age or older.

▶ The exerciser's aims and objectives should help to determine how long, how hard, and how often to exercise.

▶ A warm-up period prior to exercise is needed to raise muscle temperature, gently raise the heart rate, and to stretch the muscles and joints.

▶ Static stretching techniques are preferred to dynamic (ballistic) stretching.

▶ Intensity refers to the amount of energy expended per bout of exercise.

▶ Intensity can be monitored by perceived exertion or target heart rate.

▶ For the development of fitness, the ACSM recommends an intensity level equal to 60% to 90% of the HR max.

▶ The Karvonen Method for determining the target heart rate uses the resting heart rate and the cardiac reserve.

▶ The most common sites for taking pulse rate are the radial artery at the wrist and the carotid artery at the side of the neck.

▶ The ACSM recommends that aerobic exercise be performed 3 to 5 times per week.

▶ Exercise that is too hard, too long, or performed too often can lead to staleness.

▶ The ACSM recommends that exercise should last a minimum of 30 minutes most days of the week.

▶ The muscles, systems, and organs used in any given activity are the ones that adapt and they do so in the specific way in which they are used.

▶ Five minutes of light activity to prevent the pooling of blood in the veins is imperative during the cool-down period after exercise.

▶ Walking shoes should contain certain features if walking is to be enjoyable and safer.

▶ Walking is a low impact activity because both feet never leave the ground simultaneously.

▶ Walking is a very efficient form of locomotion except at the higher speeds. The faster one walks, the more calories one burns.

▶ The energy expenditure of walking can be increased safely by vigorously swinging the arms and by walking up hills.

▶ Walking contributes to the development of physical fitness and the enhancement of health status.

▶ Jogging shoes are a must because they are constructed to help dissipate the forces generated on impact with the ground.

▶ The energy cost of jogging for a particular body weight is about the same regardless of speed.

▶ The net caloric cost of jogging one mile is twice that of walking one mile on level ground at moderate speeds.

▶ When jogging, overstriding should be avoided. Overstriding occurs when the ankle is forward of the knee upon landing. The foot acts as a brake and stresses the knee joint.

▶ Joggers step between 600 and 750 times per mile.

▶ Joggers learn to make adjustments that dissipate the forces associated with landing.

▶ REFERENCES

1. American College of Sports Medicine. *Guidelines for Exercise Testing and Prescription*, Philadelphia: Lea and Febiger, 1991.

2. Barnard, R. J. et al. "Cardiovascular Responses to Sudden Strenuous Exercise — Heart Rate, Blood Pressure, and ECG," *Journal of Applied Physiology*, 34: (1973), p. 833.

3. de Vries, H. A. and Housh, T. J. *Physiology of Exercise*, Madison, WI: Brown and Benchmark, 1994.

4. American College of Sports Medicine, "The Recommended Quantity and Quality of Exercise for Developing and Maintaining Cardiorespiratory and Muscular Fitness in Healthy Adults," *Medicine in Science and Sport* 22: (April, 1990), p. 265.

5. American College of Sports Medicine. *Guidelines for Exercise Testing and Prescription*.

6. "An Easy-To-Swallow Prescription." *University of California at Berkeley Wellness Letter*, 10, Issue 2: (November, 1993), p. 6.

7. American College of Sports Medicine, "The Recommended Quantity and Quality of Exercise for Developing and Maintaining Cardiorespiratory and Muscular Fitness in Healthy Adults."

8. "The 10-Minute Shape-Up" *The Walking Magazine*, 6: (March/April 1991), p. 14.

9. Paffenbarger, R. S. et al. "The Association of Changes In Physical Activity Level and Other Lifestyle Characteristics With Mortality Among Men," *The New England Journal of Medicine*, 328: (February 25, 1993), p. 538.

10. White, T. P. *The Wellness Guide to Lifelong Fitness*, Rebus, N.Y.: Random House, 1993.

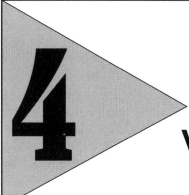

Physiological Adaptations to Walking and Jogging

A number of physiological adjustments occur as the body shifts gears from rest to physical exercise. Physical exertion requires prompt physiological and metabolic adaptations to meet the increase in energy demand. These adaptations are differentiated into two categories according to response and effect. The first category, the acute effects, are temporary and occur during and after every bout of exercise. They occur to exercisers regardless of whether they are trained or untrained. Normal physiology and metabolism are regained during the recovery period following the workout. The length of the recovery period will vary according to the exerciser's fitness level, the intensity, and the duration of the workout.

The second category, the chronic effects (also known as the "training effect") are long-lasting and accumulate as exercise is performed consistently over weeks, months, and years. The training effects become evident during the first couple of months of exercise and improvement in fitness continues for many years. Both the acute and chronic effects will be identified and explained in this chapter.

Walking and jogging are often performed outdoors so it is important to become acquainted with the environmental conditions that increase the risk of outdoor exercise. These will be covered in a fair amount of detail in this chapter.

ACUTE ADAPTATIONS (Temporary Effects)

Acute adaptations to walking and jogging refer to those physiological changes that occur after a single bout of exercise. It is important to recognize these adjustments and understand that they are temporary. Some selected acute physiological changes will be discussed.

Heart Rate

The heart's response to walking and jogging is immediate and dynamic. The rate of beating increases with the first few strides and continues to do so until a steady state has been achieved. Steady state (leveling off of heart rate) only occurs when the intensity of the workout is within the individual's capacity. It represents a period during jogging or fast walking when the oxygen demand of the activity can be supplied by the body on a minute-by-minute basis. This is the essence of an aerobic workout. The term aerobic literally means "with oxygen." Any activity is aerobic if participants can perform at a comfortable pace (mild to moderately vigorous) so that they can supply the oxygen (O_2) needed during performance. This is referred to as "steady state" exercise. The O_2 demand of exercise and O_2 supplied by the body are in balance when steady state is achieved.

Steady state cannot be attained for very vigorous exercise because the O_2 requirements exceed the exerciser's ability to supply it while exercise is in progress. This type of high intensity exercise is anaerobic which literally means "without oxygen." Anaerobic exercise can be sustained for only a few seconds. Walking and jogging are aerobic exercises; sprinting is an anaerobic exercise. High speed walking and jogging are anaerobic for people who are not trained to perform at these levels. This text emphasizes the aerobic aspects of walking and jogging because this is an effective and safe approach to enhancing health and improving cardiorespiratory fitness for the majority of adults of all ages.

Aerobic exercises require an increase in blood flow to the exercising muscles. The increase in heart rate with exercise is one of the major mechanisms for accommodating the muscle's demand for blood.

Stroke Volume

Stroke volume (SV) refers to the amount of blood that the heart can eject in one beat. The size of the stroke volume is dependent upon the amount of blood returning to the heart, the dimensions of the systemic pumping chamber (left ventricle), and the force of the contraction. Stroke volume rises linearly; that is, it is positively correlated with increases in workload up to forty to sixty percent of capacity and then levels off.[1] From this point on, further increases in blood flow occur as the result of increases in heart rate. The higher stroke volume of trained people represents one of the major differences between them and the untrained and accounts for their ability to sustain endurance activities. Figure 4.1 shows the relationship between

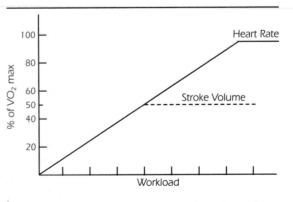

Figure 4.1 Heart rate and stroke volume responses to maximum exercise.

Table 4.1   *Average SV Values At Rest and During Maximum Exercise. Note that the SV amounts are given in ml and their equivalent weight in ounces are provided for a better appreciation of the effects of training.*

	UNTRAINED	TRAINED	HIGHLY TRAINED
At Rest	≤ 70 ml (2.4 oz.)	≤ 90 ml (3 oz)	≥ 130 ml (4.4 oz)
During Maximum Exertion	≤ 125 ml (4.2 oz)	≤150 ml (5.1 oz)	≥ 220 ml (7.4 oz)

≤ equal to or less than
≥ equal to or greater than

heart rate and stroke volume during maximum exercise.

Stroke volume is measured in milliliters (ml) of blood ejected per heart beat. The average resting and maximum stroke volumes for different levels of training appear in Table 4.1.

Cardiac Output

Cardiac output (Q) represents the amount of blood pumped by the heart in one minute. It is the product of heart rate and stroke volume (Q = HR × SV). The cardiac output increases as the intensity of exercise increases. Initially, it increases because both heart rate and stroke volume increase. Stroke volume levels off when exercise reaches approximately fifty percent of capacity, so further increases in cardiac output are due to elevations in heart rate.

The average value for cardiac output at rest is approximately four to six liters of blood per minute with values reaching twenty to twenty-five liters during maximal exercise. Well-conditioned athletes can achieve as much as forty liters during very high-intensity work. Cardiac output at rest and maximal exercise for the untrained, trained, and highly trained appear in Table 4.2.

Blood Flow

The body has the remarkable capacity to shunt blood to tissues that have the greatest need. For example, blood flow to the working muscles increases during physical activity. This is accomplished because blood flow to other tissues and organs such as the liver, kidneys and digestive system is reduced. In the competition for available blood, the muscles take precedence during physical activity. Blood flow to the digestive system is increased after a meal because this represents the greatest area of need. But if physical activity occurs immediately after eating, blood will be shunted away from the digestive system to the muscles. Digestion will slow down or stop depending upon the severity of the exercise. This is one of the major reasons why a workout should not begin until at least one hour after a meal.

More blood than usual is shunted to the skin during hot weather to help cool the body. The skin competes with the exercising muscles for the available blood, which results in the muscles receiving slightly less than normal. Less blood means less oxygen and nutrients for exercise and the workout becomes more difficult. This is why exercise in hot weather

Table 4.2   *Average Cardiac Output Values for Untrained, Trained, and Highly Trained People*

	UNTRAINED	TRAINED	HIGHLY TRAINED
At Rest	4 to 6 L	4 to 6 L	4 to 6 L
During Maximum Exercise	14 to 16 L	20 to 25 L	34 to 40 L

should be less vigorous and last for a shorter period of time.

Blood Pressure

Blood pressure is the force exerted by the heart as it pumps blood into the arteries. It is measured in millimeters of mercury (mmHg) with an instrument called a sphygmomanometer. Blood pressure is expressed in two values; systolic and diastolic. The systolic pressure is the pressure of the flow of blood when the heart beats. The diastolic pressure is the pressure between heart beats. A typical pressure for a young adult might be 120/70 (read as 120 over 70).

The systolic pressure rises during exercise — a normal and expected response that is due to an increase in cardiac output. Cardiac output increases to supply the blood and oxygen needed by the muscles and the organs (heart and lungs) that support exercise. The blood vessels in these tissues dilate to accept the extra blood, but their ability to dilate is limited. Since the increase in cardiac output is greater than the stretching ability of the blood vessels, the systolic blood pressure rises. The increase in systolic blood pressure during exercise should not exceed 250 mmHg.[2] Such an increase is abnormal and symptomatic of a cardiovascular problem.

The diastolic blood pressure changes very little during dynamic or aerobic exercise. The change is usually less than 20 mmHg plus or minus. A rise in the diastolic blood pressure to 120 mmHg is excessive and considered an abnormal response to exercise.[3]

Blood Volume

Fluid is removed from all areas of the body to produce the perspiration needed to cool the exerciser. Some of this fluid comes from the blood plasma, which reduces blood volume. As a result, the ratio of red blood cells to plasma volume, known as the hematocrit, increases. This increases the viscosity of the blood and inhibits the delivery of oxygen. Viscosity represents the thickness of the blood (more solids than liquid) which increases the blood's resistance to flow. The ratio of red blood cells to plasma volume returns to normal as fluids are consumed following the workout.

Respiratory Responses

The average person breathes twelve to sixteen times per minute at rest and forty times per minute during maximal exertion. Ventilation (V), the amount of air inhaled and exhaled per minute, is a product of the frequency of breathing (f) and the volume of air per breath or tidal volume (TV). At rest, the lungs typically ventilate five to six liters of air each minute. For example, fourteen breaths per minute at 0.4 liter per breath results in a ventilation rate of 5.6 liters of air/minute.

$$
\begin{aligned}
V &= f \times TV \\
&= 14 \times 0.4 \text{ liters} \\
&= 5.6 \text{ liters}
\end{aligned}
$$

Ventilation may escalate to 100 liters or more during maximal exertion. Large, well-conditioned athletes may move as much as 200 liters per minute.

The movement of large volumes of air from the lungs during exercise places a burden upon the respiratory muscles. The energy cost of breathing at rest represents one to two percent of the total oxygen consumed,[4] but during vigorous exercise the cost may increase to 15%.[5] The muscles of the chest wall that expand the rib cage, and the muscles of the diaphragm and abdomen require more O_2 to ventilate the lungs during vigorous exercise.

Two respiratory phenomena, side-stitch and second wind, remain mysteries in terms of their etiology. A side-stitch is a pain in the side that may be severe enough to stop activity. Constant pressure applied with both hands at the site of the stitch may alleviate the pain and allow continued activity. Breathing deeply while extending the arms overhead may also provide some relief.

A side-stitch is more likely to occur during jogging, but fast walking may also produce it. There is no scientific evidence to explain the cause or causes of developing a side-stitch, but current opinion indicates that the probable cause is ischemia (diminished blood flow) to the diaphragm or intercostal muscles. The diaphragm is a large dome-shaped muscle that separates the chest cavity from the abdominal cavity. It is the major respiratory muscle responsible for the inhalation of air into the lungs. The intercostal muscles, located between the ribs, alternately expand and contract the rib cage for inspiration and expiration of air into and out of the lungs.

Second wind is an adaptation in which the perceived effort of exercise appears to become considerably lessened although there is no change in the intensity level. The mechanisms involved are not completely understood but when second wind is achieved, breathing becomes less labored and participants experience a sense of comfort and well-being. Wilmore states that "it is possibly a result of more efficient circulation to the active tissues or of a more efficient metabolic process."[6]

Metabolic Responses

Metabolism increases with the inception of exercise and continues to do so in direct proportion to increases in exercise intensity. Metabolism may be measured indirectly with appropriate equipment by the amount of oxygen consumed during exercise on a treadmill, bicycle ergometer, or other similar devices. As the intensity of exercise steadily increases the individual's ability to supply the oxygen needed to keep pace will eventually plateau. This plateau represents the upper limit of endurance and is referred to as maximal oxygen consumption (VO_2 max). Also known as aerobic capacity or cardiorespiratory endurance, it defines a point where further increases in exercise intensity do not elicit further increases in oxygen consumption (see Figure 4.2).

VO_2 max represents the body's peak ability to assimilate, deliver and extract oxygen and it is considered to be the best indicator of physical fitness. It is a well-defined exercise endpoint that can be measured and reproduced accurately in the laboratory. These procedures are not generally available to the public, but fortunately field tests have been developed that correlate fairly well with the lab tests and may substitute for them. These will be discussed later in this chapter.

Body Size and O_2 Utilization

VO_2 max is measured in liters of oxygen utilized per minute. This absolute value is influenced considerably by body size. Since oxygen is needed and used by all body tissues, larger people take in and use more oxygen both at rest and during exercise. Aerobic capacity, when expressed in liters of oxygen per minute, is not conducive to comparison as it will yield false results. To eliminate the influence of size, aerobic capacity must be considered in terms of oxygen utilization per unit of body mass. This is accomplished by converting liters of oxygen to milliliters and then dividing by body weight in kilograms. For example, a 220 pound subject uses 4.5 liters of O_2 per minute during maximum exertion, while a 143 pound subject's capacity is 3.5 liters of O_2 per minute. From

This figure illustrates the difference in response to exercise between the trained and the untrained.

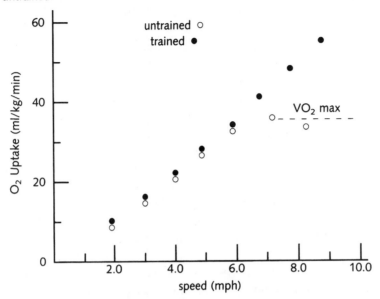

Figure 4.2 VO_2 max of trained and untrained people.

these data it appears that the larger subject is more aerobically fit due to a greater capacity to use oxygen, but observe what occurs when these values are corrected for body size. Divide body weight in pounds by 2.2 to convert to kilograms:

$$\frac{220 \text{ lbs.}}{2.2 \text{ kg.}} = 100 \text{ kg}$$

Now convert liters of O_2 per minute (LO_2/min) to milliliters of O_2 per minute by multiplying LO_2/min by 1000 (4.5 LO_2/min × 1000 = 4500 ml O_2/min). Or, you can just move the decimal point three places to the right to accomplish the same result.

Subject 1.

4.5 LO_2/min = 4500 ml. O_2/min

4500 ml. O_2/min ÷ 100 kg (220 lbs) = 45 ml. O_2/kg/min.

Subject 2.

3.5 LO_2/min = 3500 ml. O_2/min

3500 ml. O_2/min ÷ 65 kg (143 lbs) = 54 ml. O_2/kg/min.

It is obvious from this example that the lighter subject can transport, extract, and use more oxygen per unit of body mass than the larger subject and is better equipped to perform endurance activities. VO_2 max values expressed in ml O_2/kg/min. range from the mid-20s in sedentary older people to 94, which is the highest documented value recorded thus far. This enormous capacity belongs to an extremely well-conditioned male cross-country skier. The highest value recorded for female athletes is 74, also by a cross-country skier. College-age females have values in the upper thirties to low forties.

The Effects of Gender on VO$_2$ Max

Gender differences in aerobic capacity become evident after puberty with females exhibiting lower VO$_2$ values. The difference is attributed to smaller heart size per unit of body weight, less oxygen-carrying capacity due to lower blood hemoglobin concentration, less muscle tissue, and more body fat. However, there is considerable overlap between the sexes regarding aerobic capacity. World-class females competing in endurance events are aerobically superior to most males but they have lower values than world class male competitors. The differences between males and females are probably a combination of true physiological limitations and cultural restraints that have been placed upon females regarding endurance training and competition. The influence of culture and biology on female performance will eventually become clearer as more females train and compete during the next decade.

The Effects of Age on VO$_2$ max

The decline in VO$_2$ max seems to parallel the functional losses as people age. Less than 50 percent of this loss is due to the aging process, with the remainder due to an inactive lifestyle. Maximum heart rate, cardiac output, and metabolism decrease during the adult years. Body composition changes as muscle tissue is lost, thus decreasing the body's energy-producing machinery. An increase in fat tissue is an impediment to physical performance. Breathing capacity decreases as the thoracic cage (chest) loses some of its elasticity caused by weakened intercostal muscles (muscles between the ribs), increased residual volume (air remaining in the lungs after expiration), and increased rigidity of lung structures. These changes can be significantly delayed by consistent participation in exercise and physical activity.[7]

O$_2$ Deficit/O$_2$ Debt

When exercise begins, a short interval of time is needed for the body to adjust to the increased oxygen demand. This period when the oxygen demand of exercise exceeds the body's transport capability is referred to as the oxygen deficit (see Figure 4.3).

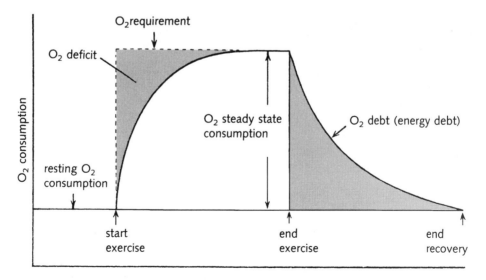

Figure 4.3   The O² deficit / O² debt.

A second phenomenon — oxygen debt — occurs during both aerobic and anaerobic exercise (see Figure 4.3). Oxygen debt refers to the amount of oxygen consumed during the exercise recovery period above that normally consumed while at rest. It is measured at the end of exercise and includes the oxygen deficit. During anaerobic exercise, the body cannot supply all the oxygen needed, resulting in a deficiency between supply and demand that must be repaid at the end of exercise. A ten-second sprint or running up two or three flights of stairs elevates heart rate and ventilation. Both persist for a few moments following the activity before gradually returning to resting levels. The extra oxygen consumed during this interval represents the oxygen debt. Aerobic exercise also produces an oxygen debt that may be entirely due to the oxygen deficit, particularly in low-intensity exercise. Aerobic exercise in excess of 50 percent of the aerobic capacity will produce lactic acid and a further increase in oxygen debt.

CHRONIC ADAPTATIONS (Training Effects)

The chronic adaptations, also referred to as the long-term effects, are those physiological and psychological changes that are the result of training. These changes represent the training effect that is gradually developed after repeated bouts of exercise.

Heart Rate

A few months of fast walking or jogging will produce a decrease in the resting heart rate (RHR) by ten to twenty-five beats per minute. The decrease in resting heart rate is accompanied by a decline in exercise heart rate for a given workload. For example, a jogging speed which elicits a heart rate of 150 beats per minute prior to training may invoke a heart rate of 125 beats per minute after a few months of training. Five to six months of training will lower the submaximum exercise heart rate by twenty to forty beats per minute. Also, the exercise heart rate returns to the resting level more rapidly as physical fitness improves.

The importance of lowered resting and exercise heart rates is that this allows more time for filling the ventricles with blood to be pumped to all of the body's tissues and more time for the delivery of oxygen and nutrients to the heart muscle. The delivery of these substances occurs during diastole (resting phase of the heart cycle) because relaxation of the heart muscle allows the coronary vessels to open up and receive the blood that it needs. Training substantially prolongs the heart's diastolic phase. The net result is that the heart operates more efficiently and with longer periods of rest.

Stroke Volume

Stroke volume and heart rate are inversely related at rest; as stroke volume increases heart rate decreases. The heart rate at rest and for a given workload is less because of the heart's enhanced ability to pump more blood per beat. This is accomplished because of more complete filling of the left ventricle combined with an increase in the contractile strength of its muscular walls, resulting in a more powerful contraction and greater emptying of the blood in the chamber. This stronger, more efficient heart is capable of meeting circulatory challenges with less beats at rest and during submaximum exercise.

Cardiac Output

Post-training cardiac output is increased considerably during maximum exercise, but there is little change during rest or submaximum work primarily because the trained individual is able to extract more oxygen from the blood. The oxygen concentration in arterial blood is essentially unchanged but the extraction rate (a-vO$_2$ difference) may be increased significantly. With training the a-vO$_2$ difference is increased, resulting in more oxygen being used as reflected by less oxygen in the venous blood.

Blood Pressure

Some controversy exists regarding the effect of exercise in reducing essential hypertension (high blood pressure, the causes of which are unknown). Essential hypertension comprises 90% to 95% of all cases of high blood pressure. Most of the evidence suggests that aerobic forms of exercise seem to be the most effective in reducing blood pressure.[8]

At this point, at least three generalizations about the relationship between exercise and blood pressure are supported by research: (1) very sedentary people tend to get the most benefit from exercise with regard to lowering the blood pressure, (2) exercise seems to be slightly more effective in lowering the blood pressure of women, and (3) heavier people tend to have smaller reductions in the systolic blood pressure than lighter people unless they lose weight simultaneously.[9]

The mechanisms by which exercise may lower blood pressure involve the hormones epinephrine and norepinephrine and their effect on resistance to blood flow in the arteries. Both hormones are vasoconstrictors that decrease the diameters of the arterioles (the smallest arteries). Sixteen weeks of aerobic exercise reduced the blood level of norepinephrine and also reduced the blood pressure.[10]

The resistance to blood flow — or peripheral resistance — is another major contributor to blood pressure. The diameter of the arterioles is largely responsible for peripheral resistance. The relationship between the two is inverse, so that the larger the diameters of the arterioles the less peripheral resistance, and the smaller the diameters the greater the resistance. Three days of aerobic exercise per week decreased peripheral resistance by 18 percent, while daily exercise resulted in a decrease of 24 percent.[11] Plasma norepinephrine levels, peripheral resistance, and blood pressure decreased as exercise frequency increased.

Blood Volume

Blood volume increases with endurance training. The volume change occurs from a significant increase in the amount of plasma (the liquid portion of the blood) and a lesser increase in blood solids (primarily the number of red blood cells). The increase in plasma volume versus red blood cells is disproportionate. The greater increase in plasma volume results in less viscous blood that is thinner (more watery). This is an important adaptation to training because thinner blood can be circulated more efficiently and with less resistance.

A trained person's red cell count is usually below average, causing the individual to appear to be anemic. In reality, trained people have a higher absolute number of red blood cells than untrained people, but on a relative basis, because of the expanded plasma volume, the numbers appear to be low. The average hematocrit (the ratio of red blood cells to plasma volume) of the general public is 40 percent to 50 percent, with males having slightly higher values (more red blood cells per unit of blood) than females. The lower hematocrit of trained people not only is an important adaptation for endurance performance but also represents a healthy change. The ideal hematocrit for running a marathon is about 50 percent, but for health it is probably closer to 40 percent for men and 35 percent for women.[12]

Heart Volume

The heart reacts to persistent walking or jogging in much the same manner as the other muscles of the body. It becomes stronger and oftentimes, larger. The volume as well as the weight of the heart increases with endurance training. Bed rest produces the opposite effect; the heart shrinks in size.

In the not-so-distant past, exercise-induced changes in the heart were considered to be pathological. The term "athlete's heart" was assigned to describe the cardiac hypertrophy (heart enlargement) seen in many athletes, and the connotation was that such a heart was harmful to health and longevity. Today, the medical community accepts these changes as normal responses to endurance training that have no long-term detrimental effects. In fact, it would be beneficial to maintain such a heart for as long as possible. Six months of inactivity following a training program will reduce heart weight and size to pretraining levels. The atrophy associated with inactivity is unavoidable.

Respiratory Responses

Some training-induced adaptations also occur in the respiratory system. The muscles that support breathing improve in both strength and endurance. This increases the amount of air that can be expired after a maximum inspiration (vital capacity) and decreases the amount of air remaining in the lungs (residual volume). Ventilation decreases slightly for a given workload and increases significantly during maximum exercise as a result of training. This indicates an improvement in the efficiency of the system. The depth of each breath (tidal volume) also increases during vigorous exercise.

Training increases blood flow in the lungs. In the sitting or standing position, many of the pulmonary capillaries in the upper regions of the lungs close down because gravity pulls blood down to the lower portions of the lungs. Exercise forces blood into the upper lobes and creates a greater surface area for the diffusion of oxygen from the alveoli (air sacs) to the pulmonary blood. Perfusion of the upper lobes of the lungs is improved with training.

Metabolic Responses

Training the Aerobic System

Endurance training improves aerobic capacity (VO_2 max) by 5 percent to 25 percent. The magnitude of the increase is dependent primarily upon the initial level of fitness. Those who are the least fit make the most improvement simply because they are furthest away from their genetic potential.[13]

Fitness gains come rather quickly during the first few months of training, with further increases occurring in smaller increments as fitness improves until VO_2 max reaches its peak. VO_2 max is reached with six months to two years of training.

The improvement in VO_2 max is caused by a combination of physiological adaptations. First, the number and size of mitochondria increase. The mitochondria (often referred to as the cells' powerhouse) are organelles within the cells that utilize oxygen to produce the ATP needed by the muscles. ATP (adenosine triphosphate) is a high-energy compound that provides the fuel that the body uses. Second, enzymes located within the mitochondria that accelerate the chemical reactions needed for the production of ATP are increased. These increases in the mitochondria and their enzymes produce greater amounts of energy and improvement in physical fitness. Third, there is an increase in maximal cardiac output and local blood supply in the exercising muscles. Fourth, more oxygen is extracted from the blood by the exercising muscles. At rest, the arteries carry approximately 20 ml O_2 per 100 ml of blood. The veins carry about 14 ml O_2 per 100 ml of blood. When the oxygen value in the veins is subtracted from the oxygen value in the arteries, it yields the amount of oxygen used by the body. This value is termed the arterial-venous oxygen difference (a–vO_2 diff), and at rest it is equal to 6 ml O_2/100 ml blood. Since exercise increases the body's need for oxygen, the extraction rate increases and the a-vO_2 difference widens. Training increases the a-vO_2 difference during maximum exercise but may not increase it at rest or during submaximum exercise.

The Effect of Aging on the Aerobic System

Aerobic capacity decreases with age, but it decreases more slowly for people who are physically fit. Researchers at San Diego State University studied the effect of exercise on 15 men who walked, jogged, swam, and cycled 3 to 4 days per week for 23 years.[14] The men averaged 45 years of age at the start of the study and 68 years at the 23-year mark. Their VO_2 max declined 13 percent during 23 years, compared to an amazing 41 percent decline for a nonexercising group of men of similar age. The average VO_2 max as people age is a gradual but systematic 1 percent per year. The researchers concluded that the 13% loss in VO_2 max for the exercise group represented a true effect of aging. If the aging effect (13% decline) is factored out of the decline experienced by the nonexercisers, two thirds of their decrease in VO_2 max is due to inactivity rather than aging.

This important long-term study has provided evidence to support what many exercisers and researchers by logical deduction and anecdotal evidence already knew — that physical training delays the deterioration of aerobic capacity at least until people reach their sixties.

The Effect of Inherited Factors

Aerobic capacity is finite. Each of us is endowed with an aerobic potential limited by our heredity. A small percentage of people inherit the potential to achieve amazing feats of endurance, as exemplified by performances in marathons, ultramarathons, Iron Man Triathalons, cross-country runs lasting weeks or months, and long-distance bike races. Most of us are in the average category for aerobic capacity, but all of us can achieve our potential with endurance training.

Researchers have attempted to quantify the influence of heredity as a component of VO_2 max. In other words, how much of the variability seen among people in VO_2 max is due to inherited factors? Although this line of inquiry is yet to be fully resolved, the differences observed among identical twins, fraternal twins, and other siblings have provided some clues. The best available evidence suggests that the genetic component represents 40% of the known factors regarding the achievable VO_2 max for any individual. Those who have inherited superior cardiorespiratory endowment have the physical structure to benefit maximally from training and may become national or world-class performers provided they train diligently and intelligently. Those who are endowed to a lesser extent (the majority of people) also benefit from training. They may not have the foundation to become high-level competitors, but they can train to their potential and enjoy their own accomplishments.

The Anaerobic Threshold (Onset of Blood Lactic Acid)

Even though VO_2 max reaches a peak early in the training program, aerobic performance continues to improve for many years with harder and continued training. The question, then, is, how can physical performance continue to improve after VO_2 max has leveled off? This question can be answered with an example. Let us assume that a female jogger has achieved her aerobic potential of 54 ml/kg/min with two years of regular training. At this point, she is able to jog a five-mile course at 38 ml/kg/min, or 70 percent of her aerobic capacity. After two more years of vigorous training (VO_2 max still at 54 ml/kg/min), she is now able to sustain 47 ml/kg/min pace for the same distance, or 88 percent of her aerobic capacity. The past two years of training have permitted her to use more oxygen, thereby sustaining a faster pace for the course without dipping materially into the anaerobic fuel systems that produce lactic acid and oxygen debt.

The point during exercise where blood lactate suddenly begins to increase is defined as the anaerobic threshold and is also known as "the onset of blood lactate accumulation." Training moves the anaerobic threshold closer to the VO_2 max, allowing people to exercise at a higher percentage of their capacity before lactic acid accumulates to the point where it begins to interfere with muscle contraction and physical performance. Two people with the same VO_2 max will perform differently in an endurance event if one has an anaerobic threshold substantially higher than the other.

DECONDITIONING — LOSING THE TRAINING EFFECT

Deconditioning takes place when training is discontinued or significantly reduced. E. F. Coyle investigated the physiological changes that accompany detraining as well as the approximate timetable of their occurrence.[15] The subjects in this study had been actively training for ten years. They abandoned training for 84 days (12 weeks) so that Coyle could observe and measure the changes that took place. Coyle noted that some systems of the body showed the effects of detraining rapidly, while others reacted more slowly. Stroke volume declined substantially in the first 12 days. As expected, the decline was accomplished by a significant reduction in aerobic capacity, which declined 16 percent by the fifty-sixth day of the deconditioning period. The oxidative enzyme level in the muscles dropped 40 percent at the end of eight weeks. However, the capillary density of the muscles declined by only 7 percent below the trained state by the end of the detraining period, and mitochondrial enzymes remained 50 percent higher than those of sedentary control subjects.

WALKING/JOGGING IN HOT AND COLD WEATHER

Human beings are compelled to function in a variety of environmental conditions. People live and work in frigid, temperate, and tropical zones, at sea level and at high altitudes and have adapted and learned to tolerate extremes in temperature. In cold weather, body temperature may be maintained by putting on more clothes or by increasing the body's production of heat through physical movement or shivering. In hot environments heat may be lost through sweating, increasing blood flow to the skin, and by wearing as little clothing as the law and culture will allow.

Humans are homeotherms (meaning "same heat") who are capable of maintaining the constant internal temperature necessary for the support of such life-sustaining processes as cellular metabolism, oxygen transport, muscular contraction, etc. We exist within a relatively narrow band of internal temperature, ranging from 97 to 99 degrees, but our temperature may (and often does) rise to 104 degrees during exercise. Temperatures that rise above 106 degrees, if not rapidly reduced, often result in cellular deterioration, permanent brain damage, and death; while temperatures below 93 degrees slow metabolism to the extent that unconsciousness and cardiac arrhythmias (disturbances of normal heart rhythm that can be fatal) are likely.

Heat is produced in the body as a by-product of metabolism. Physical activities significantly increase metabolism, so more heat than normal is generated. Heat must be dissipated effectively, or heat build-up (hyperthermia) may result in illness and possible death. Hyperthermia is abnormally high body temperature. Heat exhaustion is a serious condition but not an imminent threat to life. It is characterized by dizziness, fainting, rapid pulse, and cool skin. Treatment includes immediate cessation of activity and moving to a cool, shady place. The victim is placed in a reclining position and given cool fluids to drink.

Heat stroke is a medical emergency and a threat to life. It is the most severe of the heat-induced illnesses. The symptoms include a high temperature (106° F or above) and dry skin caused by the cessation of sweating. These symptoms are accompanied by some or all of the following: delirium, convulsions, and loss of consciousness. The early warning signs include chills, nausea, headache, and general weakness. Victims of heat stroke should be rushed immediately to the nearest hospital for treatment.

▶ MECHANISMS OF HEAT LOSS AND HEAT TRANSFER

Heat is lost from the body by conduction, radiation, convection, and evaporation of sweat.

Conduction, convection, and radiation are mechanisms responsible for heat transfer. The weather conditions determine whether walkers and joggers lose or gain heat through these mechanisms. Evaporation of sweat is a true heat loss mechanism because the transfer of heat can only travel in one direction — from the body to the environment.

Conduction

Conduction occurs when there is direct physical contact between objects as long as one of the objects is cooler than the other. The greater the difference in temperature between the objects, the greater the transfer of heat. If you enter an air-conditioned room from outdoors on a summer day and sit in a cool leather chair, you lose heat through contact with the cooler chair.

Conductive heat loss occurs even more rapidly in water. Water is not an insulator but a conductor. It absorbs several thousand times more heat than air at the same temperature. This is the reason sitting at the poolside is more comfortable than sitting in the pool, even if the temperature of both air and water are equal.

Convection

Heat loss by convection occurs when a gas or liquid that is cooler than the body moves across the skin. If the gas or liquid is warmer than skin temperature the body will accept heat rather than lose it.

Convective heat loss from the body to the environment is increased if a cool breeze is blowing, either naturally caused or caused by an electric fan, or if one is swimming in cool water. Swimming is more effective for heat loss than floating because of the flow of water over the body. Convective heat loss is augmented by conductive heat loss when one participates in water activities. The heat loss and heat transfer mechanisms do not function in isolation; they often work together to rid the body of heat.

Radiation

Heat is lost through radiation because humans, animals, and inanimate objects constantly emit heat by electromagnetic waves to cooler objects in the environment. This occurs without physical contact between objects. Heat is simply transferred on a temperature gradient from warmer objects to cooler ones.

Heat loss by radiation is very effective when the air temperature (ambient temperature) is well below skin temperature. This is one of the major reasons that outdoor exercise in cool weather is better tolerated than the same exercise in hot weather. Temperatures in the upper 80s and 90s will probably result in heat gain by radiation.

Evaporation

Evaporation of sweat is the major method of heat loss during exercise, and this process is most effective when the humidity is low. High humidity significantly impairs the evaporative process because the air is very saturated and cannot accept much more moisture. If both temperature and humidity are high, losing heat is difficult by any of these processes. Under these conditions, adjusting the intensity and duration of exercise or moving indoors where the climate can be controlled may be beneficial.

Heat loss by evaporation occurs only when the sweat on the surface of the skin is vaporized, that is, converted to a gas. The conversion of liquid to a gas at the skin level requires heat supplied by the body. Beads of sweat that roll off the body do not contribute to the cooling process — only sweat that evaporates does.

Exercise in hot and humid conditions forces the body to divert more blood than usual from the working muscles to the skin in an effort to carry the heat accumulating in the deeper recesses to the outer shell. The net result is that the exercising muscles are deprived of a full complement of blood and cannot work as long or as hard. Exercise is therefore more difficult in hot and humid weather.

Heat loss by evaporation is seriously impeded when participants wear nonporous garments such as rubberized and plastic exercise suits. These garments encourage sweating, but their nonporous nature does not allow sweat to evaporate. This practice is dangerous because it may easily result in heat buildup and dehydration (excessive water loss), leading to heat-stress illnesses. You should dress for hot-weather exercise by wearing shorts and a porous top. A mesh, baseball-type cap is optional. It is effective in blocking the absorption of radiant heat if you exercise in the middle of the day because the sun's rays are vertical. You do not need to wear a cap when exercising in the cooler parts of the day or if the sun is not shining.

GUIDELINES FOR WALKING AND JOGGING IN HOT WEATHER

Guidelines for exercising in heat and humidity have been developed for road races, but these can be applied to any strenuous physical activity performed outdoors during warm weather. Ambient conditions are considered safe when the temperature is below 70° F and the humidity is below 45%. Caution should be used when the temperature and humidity exceed these values. People who are trained and heat acclimated can continue to exercise at higher temperatures and humidities but they should take precautions to prevent heat illness. Figure 4.4 gives guidelines when temperature and humidity are factors.

Notice the relationship between temperature and humidity in Figure 4.4. The higher the percent humidity the lower the temperature must be for safe exercise conditions to exist. Conversely, the lower the humidity, the higher the temperature can be for exercise to be safe.

The keys to exercising without incident in hot weather are to acclimate to the heat and maintain the body's normal fluid level. The major consequence of dehydration (excessive fluid loss) is a reduction in blood volume.[16] This results in sluggish circulation that decreases the delivery of oxygen to the exercising muscles. Second, lowered blood volume results in less blood that can be sent to the skin to remove the heat generated by exercise. If too much of the blood volume is lost, sweating will stop and the body temperature will rise, leading to heat-stress illness. Heat illness is a serious problem that can be avoided by following a few guidelines designed to preserve the body's fluid level:

1. **Hyperhydration — pre-exercise:**

   Before walking or jogging, you should drink 12 to 20 ounces of a salted liquid 15 to 30 minutes before exercising. You can purchase a commercially prepared sports drink such as Gatorade or mix a teaspoon of salt in a gallon of lemonade. Water is not the best liquid source because it stimulates the production of urine, leaving less liquid for sweating.

2. **Fluid replacement during exercise:**

   Recommendations for replacing liquid during exercise are less clear. The primary reason for drinking during exercise is to maintain body water stores so that sweating can continue.

   a. Water is the preferred drink when exercise lasts less than 2 hours. Water exits the stomach rapidly and moves to the tissues that need it.

   b. Urine production is not a problem during exercise because fluid is used to produce sweat.

   c. A beverage containing salt and sugar is preferred if exercise lasts longer than 2 hours (for example, during marathons, long-distance cycling, and ultra-distance running events and triathalons).

   d. You should drink 6 to 8 ounces every 15 minutes during exercise.

3. **Post-exercise fluid replacement:**

   a. Plain water is a poor drink during recovery from exercise because it suppresses

Relative Humidity (%)	Temperature (°F)							Caution		Extreme Caution
	60	65	70	75	80	85	90	95	100
20	59	62	65	68	70	73	76	79	82
40	59	63	66	69	73	76	79	83	86
60	60	63	67	71	75	79	83	87	91
80	60	64	69	73	78	82	86	91	95
100	60	65	70	75	80	85	90	95	100

From D. Anspaugh, M. Hamrick, F. Rosato (1994), *Wellness Concepts and Applications,* St. Louis: Mosby. Reprinted by permission.

Figure 4.4   Guidelines for exercise in heat and humidity.

the thirst drive, so fluid intake stops before rehydration is complete.

b. You should avoid alcoholic beverages and caffeinated beverages because these stimulate urine production. All ingested fluids need to be retained for the purpose of rehydration.

c. You should drink fluids that contain salt and sugar. Again, commercial sports drinks are appropriate. In addition, they taste good which encourages exercisers to drink more. This counteracts the tendency of most people to drink less than they need if water is the alternative.

4. **Since 95% of the weight lost during exercise is fluid, weight loss becomes a good indicator of the amount of fluid loss. For estimating fluid loss you should:**

a. Weigh yourself in the nude before and after exercise.

b. Towel off sweat completely after exercise and then weigh yourself.

c. Each pound of weight loss represents about 1 pint of fluid loss. Be sure to drink that and more after exercise.

5. **Other considerations:**

a. Modify the exercise program by (1) working out during cooler times of day, (2) choosing shady routes where water is available, (3) slowing the pace and/or shortening the duration of exercise on particularly oppressive days, and (4) wearing light, loose, porous clothing to facilitate the evaporation of sweat.

b. Never take salt tablets. They are a stomach irritant, they attract fluid to the gut, they sometimes pass through the digestive system undissolved, and they may perforate the stomach lining.

c. Exercise must be prolonged, produce profuse sweating, and occur over a number of consecutive days to reduce potassium stores. For the average bout of exercise, you do not need to worry about depleting potassium or make a special effort to replace it. The daily consumption of fresh fruits and vegetables, as suggested by the new food consumption guidelines is all that is needed.

GUIDELINES FOR JOGGING AND WALKING IN COLD WEATHER

Problems related to exercise in cold weather include frostbite and hypothermia (abnormally low body temperature). Frostbite can lead to permanent damage or loss of a body part from gangrene. This can be prevented by adequately protecting exposed areas such as fingers, nose, ears, facial skin, and toes. Gloves, preferably mittens or thick socks, should be worn to protect the fingers, hands and wrists. A stocking hat is preferable for two reasons: (1) blood vessels in the scalp do not constrict effectively, so a significant amount of heat is lost if a head covering is not worn, and (2) a stocking-type hat can be pulled down to protect the ears. In very cold or windy weather, you can use surgical or ski masks and scarves to keep facial skin warm and to moisten and warm inhaled air. All exposed or poorly protected flesh is vulnerable to frostbite when the temperature is low and the wind chill high. Figure 4.5 can be used as a safety guide for working and exercising in cold, windy weather. Notice the relationship between the temperature and wind speed. A temperature of 40° F feels like 16° F if the wind is blowing at 25 mph.

People often experience a hacking cough for a minute or two after physical exertion in cold weather. This is a normal response and should not cause alarm. Very cold, dry air may not be fully moistened when it is inhaled rapidly and in large volumes during exercise. This causes the lining of the throat to dry out. When exercise is discontinued, the respiratory rate slows and the volume of inhaled air decreases, allowing enough time for the body to fully moisturize it. Coughing stops within a couple of minutes as the linings are remoistened.

Hypothermia is the most severe of the problems associated with outdoor activity in cold weather. Hypothermia occurs when body heat is lost faster than it can be produced. This can be a life-threatening situation.

Exercise in cold weather requires insulating layers of clothing to preserve normal body heat. Without this protection, body heat is quickly lost because of the large temperature gradient between the skin and environment. In addition to the insulating qualities of layers of clothing, a layer or two can be discarded if you get too hot.

Hypothermia can occur even if the air temperature is above freezing. For instance, the rate of heat loss for any temperature is influenced by wind velocity. Wind velocity increases the amount of cold air molecules that come in contact with the skin. The more cold molecules, the more effective the heat loss. The speed of walking or jogging into the wind must be added to the speed of the wind chill.

You should wear enough clothing to stay warm but not so much that you induce profuse sweating. The amount of clothing that is appropriate for outdoor activities is dependent upon the experience that comes from participation in cold weather conditions. Clothing that becomes wet with sweat loses it insulating qualities. It becomes a conductor of heat, moving it from the body quickly and potentially endangering the exerciser.

If you exercise or work outdoors in cold weather, you may want to wear polypropylene undergarments. Polypropylene is designed to whisk perspiration from the skin so that

Actual Thermometer Reading (°F)											
50	**40**	**30**	**20**	**10**	**0**	**−10**	**−20**	**−30**	**−40**	**−50**	**−60**
Wind Speed (mph)				Equivalent Temperature (°F)							
Calm	50	40	30	20	10	0	−10	−20	−30	−40	−50	−60
5	48	37	27	16	6	−5	−15	−26	−36	−47	−57	−68
10	40	28	16	4	−9	−21	−33	−46	−58	−70	−83	−95
15	36	22	9	−5	−18	−36	−45	−58	−72	−85	−99	−112
20	32	18	4	−10	−25	−39	−53	−67	−82	−96	−110	−124
25	30	16	0	−15	−29	−44	−59	−74	−88	−104	−118	−133
30	28	13	−2	−18	−33	−48	−63	−79	−94	−109	−125	−140
35	27	11	−4	−20	−35	−49	−67	−82	−98	−113	−129	−145
40*	26	10	−6	−21	−37	−53	−69	−85	−100	−116	−132	−148

Little danger (for properly clothed person)   Increasing danger — cover up fully (hands, ears, face, head)   Great danger — exercise indoors

* Wind speeds greater than 40 mph have little additional effect.
From B. J. Sharkey (1990), *Physiology of Fitness*, Champaign, IL: Human Kinetics Books. Reprinted by permission.

Figure 4.5   Wind chill index.

evaporative cooling will not rob heat from the body. You should wear a warm outer garment, preferably made of wool, over this material. If it is windy, you should wear a breathable windbreaker as the outer layer.

If you follow the guidelines for activity in hot and cold weather, you can usually participate quite comfortably all year long.

◤ ASSESSING CARDIORESPIRATORY ENDURANCE

Aerobic capacity (VO_2 max) is measured quite accurately in the laboratory with a motor-driven treadmill or bicycle ergometer along with gas collection and analysis systems. This equipment is expensive and requires considerable expertise by those doing the testing. In addition, only one subject at a time may be tested so there is a sizeable investment in time. These procedures are inappropriate for large groups; therefore, investigators have attempted to find economical substitutes that would yield accurate results. Three field tests have been selected in lieu of laboratory tests. They correlate quite well with the laboratory tests and are easier to administer.

◤ WALKING TESTS

The Rockport Fitness Walking Test*

Directions

This walking test estimates aerobic capacity based on the variables of age, gender, time required to walk 1 mile, and the heart rate

---

*Reprinted by permission of The Rockport Company, Inc. © (1993) The Rockport Company, Inc. All Rights Reserved.

achieved at the end of the test. The guidelines for taking the test are as follows:

1. Heart rate is counted for 15 seconds and multiplied by 4 to get beats per minute.
2. The course should be flat and measured, preferably a 440-yard track.
3. Use a stop watch or a watch with a second hand.
4. Warm up for 5 to 10 minutes before taking the test. Preparation for the test should include a 1/4 mile walk followed by stretching exercises.
5. During the test the walk should be a brisk pace and 1 mile should be covered as rapidly as possible.
6. Take your pulse rate immediately after the test. This rate should then be marked on the chart on the following pages that is appropriate for your age and gender.
7. Draw a vertical line through your time and a horizontal line through your heart rate. The point where the lines intersect determines your fitness level (see the charts on the following pages).

Rockport provides a series of 20-week walking-for-fitness programs that are based on the results of the walking test. These may be obtained for a nominal fee ($1.00 at this writing) by sending a request to Rockport Fitness Walking Test, 72 Howe St. Marlboro, Massachusetts, 01752.

These charts are designed to tell you how fit you are compared with other individuals of your age and gender. For example, if your coordinates place you in the "above average" section of the chart, you are in better shape than the average person in your category.

The charts are based on weights of 170 lb for men and 125 lb for women. If you weigh substantially more, your relative cardiovascular fitness level will be slightly overestimated. If you weigh substantially less, your relative cardiovascular level will be slightly underestimated.

Tables 4.3 through 4.7 are for Males Only

20 to 29 Year-Old Males

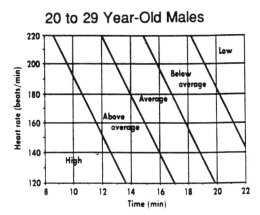

Table 4.3

30 to 39 Year-Old Males

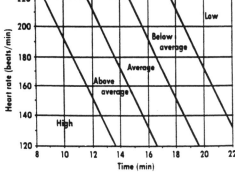

Table 4.4

40 to 49 Year-Old Males

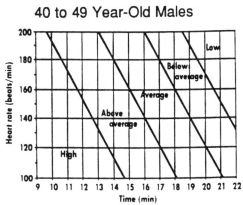

Table 4.5

50 to 59 Year-Old Males

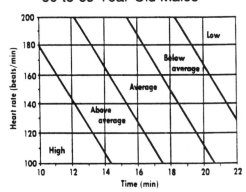

Table 4.6

60 Year-Old and Older Males

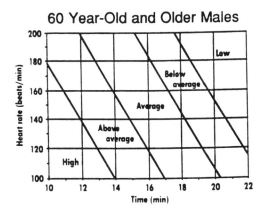

Table 4.7

▶ Tables 4.8 through 4.12 are for Females Only

20 to 29 Year-Old Females

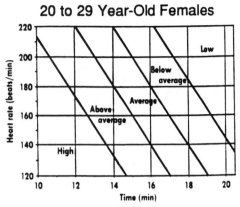

Table 4.8

30 to 39 Year-Old Females

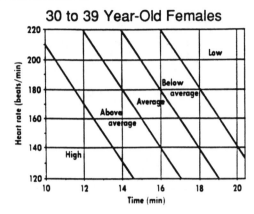

Table 4.9

40 to 49 Year-Old Females

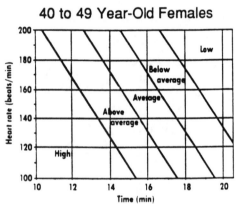

Table 4.10

50 to 59 Year-Old Females

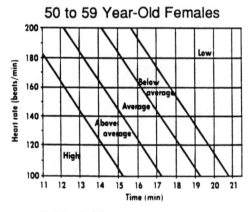

Table 4.11

60 Year-Old and Older Females

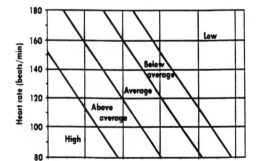

Table 4.12

The 3-Mile Walking Test

Directions

This is a 3-mile test to fatigue; no running is allowed. The length of this test and the fact that it demands a maximum effort (walking the distance as quickly as you can) requires you to train for at least 6 weeks before making the attempt. Students make their best scores when they are allowed two practice trials walking the distance. This experience enables them to find the pace that will result in the fastest time within their fitness capacity.

Suggestions for taking the test include the following:

1. Walk at an even pace, but attempt the fastest pace that you can maintain for the entire distance.

2. Avoid starting out too fast — if you do, you will run out of energy too soon.

3. Rest the day before and the day after the test.

4. Eat a predominantly carbohydrate meal (e.g., pasta, rice, potatoes, pancakes) that is low in fat. Select foods that have given you no digestive problems in the past. Eat this approximately 2 to 3 hours before the test.

5. Be sure to drink plenty of liquids the day of the test. Water, Gatorade, and fruit juices diluted with half water are appropriate.

6. Warm up before the test. About 5 to 6 minutes of walking followed by stretching exercises will suffice.

7. Cool down after the test by walking at a slower pace for 5 to 6 minutes and do the same stretching exercises as you performed in the warm-up period.

The test is best administered on a running track that is 1/4 mile long; 12 full laps around will complete the test. After completing the test, record your time and compare it with the numbers listed in Table 4.13 to determine your fitness level. For example, a 19-year old female walks the 3 miles in 41 minutes and 28 seconds (41:28). Her fitness level is "Fair."

JOGGING/RUNNING TEST

The 1.5 Mile Test

Cooper found that the 1.5 mile run correlated very highly with treadmill tests in the measurement of aerobic capacity. It has the following advantages over laboratory testing: (1) a number of subjects can be tested at the same time, (2) it is easy to administer, and (3) the only equipment needed is a measured course and a stopwatch.

The validity and accuracy of the 1.5 mile test can be increased by allowing the subjects an

Table 4.13   Level of Aerobic Fitness — 3-Mile Walking Test

Fitness Category	13–19 Yr Male	13–19 Yr Female	20–29 Yr Male	20–29 Yr Female	30–39 Yr Male	30–39 Yr Female
Excellent	<33:00	<35:00	<34:00	<36:00	<35:00	<37:50
Good	33–37:30	35–39:30	34–38:30	36–40:30	35–40:00	37:30–42:00
Fair	37:31–41:00	39:31–43:00	38:31–42:00	40:31–44:00	40:01–44:30	42:01–46:30
Poor	41:01–45:00	43:01–47:00	42:01–46:00	44:01–48:00	44:31–49:00	46:31–51:00
Very Poor	>45:00	>47:00	>46:00	>48:00	>49:00	>51:00

< = Less than; > = greater than.

From D. Anspaugh, M. Hamrick, F. Rosato (1994), *Wellness Concepts and Applications,* St. Louis: Mosby. Reprinted by permission.

opportunity to have several practice trials over the test course spaced over a week or ten days. Thus, each subject becomes familiar with the course and with the pace required to produce an optimal score. After several practice trials have been allowed, each subject should attempt to run the course in the fastest possible time within his/her capacity. The most valid results are attained when subjects make an all-out effort.

The time required to cover the distance represents the score earned. Walking is allowed if one needs to rest, but of course, it will detract from the score since it adds time to cover the distance. Table 4.14 translates the time taken to cover the distance into one's estimated aerobic capacity (VO_2 max). After obtaining this value, refer to Table 4.15 for placement into a fitness category. For example, a 22 year old female covers the 1.5 mile distance in 13:20. Table 4.14 indicates that this female has an estimated VO_2 max of 37 ml/kg/min. Table 4.15 indicates that 37 ml/kg/min falls in the "fair" category but note that the average VO_2 max of females is 15% to 20% lower than that of males. Therefore, to correctly assess this female's fitness level you must shift one category to the left so that she moves from "fair" to "average." No adjustment is needed in Table 4.15 to correctly assess the fitness level of males.

Table 4.14 An Estimate of Aerobic Capacity

Time in Minutes and Seconds	Estimated VO_2 max in ml/kg/min
7:30 or less	75
7:31– 8:00	72
8:01– 8:30	67
8:31– 9:00	62
9:01– 9:30	58
9:31–10:00	55
10:01–10:30	52
10:31–11:00	49
11:01–11:30	46
11:31–12:00	44
12:01–12:30	41
12:31–13:00	39
13:01–13:30	37
13:31–14:00	36
14:01–14:30	34
14:31–15:00	33
15:01–15:30	31
15:31–16:00	30
16:01–16:30	28
16:31–17:00	27
17:01–17:30	26
17:31–18:00	25

Adapted from K. H. Cooper. "A Means of Assessing Maximal Oxygen Intake," *Journal of The American Medical Association* 203 (1968): 201–204. Reprinted by permission.

Table 4.15 Fitness Levels for the 1½ Mile Jog/Run Test

Age Group (yrs)	High	Good	Average	Fair	Poor
10–19	Above 66	57–66	47–56	38–46	Below 38
20–29	Above 62	53–62	43–52	33–42	Below 33
30–39	Above 58	49–58	39–48	30–38	Below 30
40–49	Above 54	45–54	36–44	26–35	Below 26
50–59	Above 50	42–50	34–41	24–33	Below 24
60–69	Above 46	39–46	31–38	22–30	Below 22
70–79	Above 42	36–42	28–35	20–27	Below 20

The average maximal O_2 uptake of females is 15 to 20 percent lower than that of males. To find the appropriate category for females, locate the score in the above table and shift one category to the left, e.g., the "Average" category for males is the "Good" category for females.

Adapted from Jack H. Wilmore. *Training for Sport and Activity* (Boston: Allyn and Bacon, Inc., 1982). Reprinted by permission.

Summary

- The acute adaptations to exercise refer to those physiological changes that occur during and after a single about of exercise.

- Heart rate and stroke volume rise linearly for exercise of increasing intensity, but stroke volume levels off at approximately 50% of max capacity.

- Cardiac output increases during maximum exercise as the result of training.

- The body shunts blood to areas of greatest need — to the muscles during exercise, to the digestive system after a meal, etc.

- The systolic blood pressure rises during exercise. This is a normal response due to the rise in cardiac output.

- The viscosity of the blood increases during heavy exercise of prolonged duration.

- The energy cost of breathing during rest is about one to two percent of the oxygen consumed but during vigorous exercise the cost may increase to 15%.

- Aerobic capacity (VO_2 max) is the body's peak ability to assimilate, deliver, and extract oxygen for physical work.

- Males generally have higher aerobic capacities than females.

- VO_2 max decreases with age but age per se is responsible for less than 50% of the decline — inactivity is responsible for the majority of the loss.

- Training reduces the resting heart rate and increases the resting and maximum stroke volume.

- Training reduces the resting blood pressure for most people.

- Training reduces the viscosity of the blood by increasing the plasma volume.

- Heart volume increases with aerobic training.

- Aerobic capacity can be improved by 5% to 25% with aerobic training.

- Inherited factors are responsible for approximately 40% of our achieved aerobic capacity.

- The systems of the body decondition at various rates when training ceases.

- Heat is lost from the body by conduction, convection, radiation, and evaporation.

- The keys to exercising safely in high heat and humidity are to acclimate to the heat and to be adequately hydrated.

- The most common cold-related exercise injury is frostbite; the most serious cold weather injury is hypothermia.

▶ REFERENCES

1. Wilmore, J. H. and Costill, D. L. *Training for Sport and Activity*, Dubuque, Iowa: Wm. C. Brown, 1988.

2. American College of Sports Medicine. *Guidelines for Exercise Testing and Prescription*, Philadelphia: Lea and Febiger, 1991.

3. American College of Sports Medicine, *Guidelines for Exercise Testing*.

4. de Vries, H. A. and Housh, T. J. *Physiology of Exercise*, Madison: WCB Brown and Benchmark, 1994.

5. McArdle, W. D., Katch, F. I., and Katch, V. L. *Exercise Physiology*, Philadelphia: Lea and Febiger, 1991.

6. Wilmore, J. H., et al.

7. Williams, M. H. *Lifetime Fitness and Wellness*, Madison CB Brown and Benchmark, 1993.

8. Massie, B. M. "To Combat Hypertension, Increase Activity," *The Physician and Sportsmedicine* 20, No. 5: (May, 1992), p. 88.

9. Hagburg, J. M. "Exercise Fitness, and Hypertension," in C. Bouchard et al. (Eds.), *Exercise, Fitness and Health: A Consensus of Current Knowledge*, Champaign, IL: Human Kinetics, 1990.

10. Duncan, J. J. et al. "The Effects of Aerobic Exercise on Plasma Catecholamines and Blood Pressure In Patients with Mild Essential Hypertension," *Journal of the American Medical Association*, 254: (1985), p. 2609.

11. Nelson, L. et al. "Effect of Changing Levels of Physical Activity on Blood-Pressure and Hemodynamics in Essential Hypertension," *Lancet*, 11: (1986), p. 473.

12. "What's the Ideal Hematocrit?," *The Physician and Sportsmedicine*, 18, No. 8: (August, 1990) p. 35.

13. Rosato, F. D. *Fitness for Wellness — The Physical Connection*, St. Paul: West Publishing Co., 1994.

14. Kasch, F. W. et al., "The Effects of Physical Activity and Inactivity On Aerobic Power in Older Men (A Longitudinal Study)," *The Physician and Sportsmedicine* 18, No 4: (April, 1990), p. 73.

15. Cole, E. F. et al. "Effects of Detraining On Responses to Submaximal Exercise," *Journal of Applied Physiology*, 59: (1985), p. 853.

16. Stamford, B. J. "How To Avoid Dehydration," *The Physician and Sportsmedicine*, 18, No. 7: (July, 1990), p. 135.

Reducing the Risk of Cardiovascular Disease: The Role of Exercise

The health benefits associated with walking and jogging, as well as other aerobic exercises, have been systematically researched during the last couple of decades. The evidence supporting health enhancement through consistent participation in physical exercise has been accumulating steadily.

This chapter focuses on the effect of exercise in preventing, delaying, and to a lesser extent, treating coronary heart disease. To this end, the emphasis is on the modifying effect that exercise has on the risk factors for coronary heart disease.

CARDIOVASCULAR DISEASES

Cardiovascular diseases — diseases of the heart and blood vessels — are the leading causes of death in the United States. They are responsible for approximately 44% of the total number of deaths that occur annually.[1] Sixty-nine million Americans have one or more forms of cardiovascular disease and nearly one million of them die each year. The leading form of cardiovascular disease, claiming nearly 500,000 lives annually, is coronary heart disease. This form of the disease is characterized by the accumulation of plaque in the blood vessels that supply the heart with oxygen and nutrients. The build-up of plaque, referred to as atherosclerosis, can lead to a heart attack. The medical term for a heart attack is myocardial infarction.

Coronary heart disease is the classic type of heart attack that occurs when obstructions (blood clots) or spasms (constricture of coronary vessels) disrupt the flow of blood to a portion of the heart muscle. The site of obstruction or spasm determines the extent of muscle damage. Heart attacks of any magnitude result in irreversible injury and heart muscle death. The dead muscle forms scar tissue that no longer contributes to the heart's ability to pump blood. The heart becomes a less efficient pump after a heart attack. If the attack is massive, and causes extensive damage, the heart and its host will die.

Atherosclerosis is the primary cause of coronary heart disease. It is a slow progressive disease of large and mid-sized arteries. Atherosclerosis is the process in which fatty substances, cholesterol, calcium, fibrin, and cellular debris form plaques that obstruct the flow of blood. If left unchecked plaques continue to enlarge until the arterial channels narrow significantly, creating the environment for blood clots or spasms to occur at these sites of disease. If blood flow is completely impeded a heart attack will occur and muscle tissue damage will follow. See Figures 5.1 and 5.2.

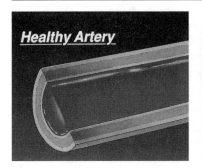
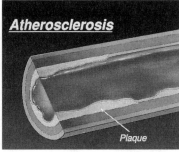
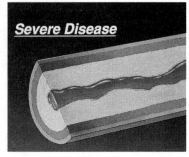

From *Heart of a Healthy Life*. Courtesy of the American Heart Association, © 1992.

Figure 5.1   Plaque build-up during various stages of atherosclerosis.

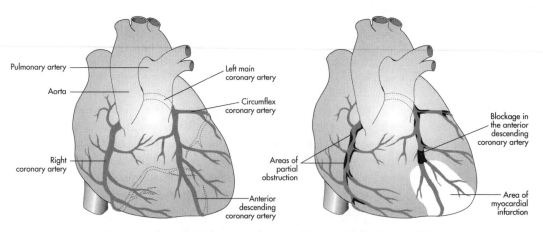

From W. W. K. Hoeger, *Principles and Labs for Physical Fitness and Wellness*, 3d ed. Englewood, CO: Morton Publishing Co., 1994.

Figure 5.2   Heart attack caused by a blood clot.

RISK FACTORS
FOR HEART DISEASE

Although most heart attacks occur later in the life cycle (55% after the age of 65) the processes responsible for them begin quite early, often before adolescence. The processes that lead to atherosclerosis and coronary heart disease are referred to as cardiovascular risk factors. They were identified in the landmark Framingham Heart Disease Study which began in 1949 and continues today. The risk factors are genetic or learned behaviors that increase the probability of premature illness and death from coronary heart disease. The American Heart Association (AHA) categorizes the risk factors in the following manner: (1) major risk factors that cannot be changed — increasing age, male gender, and heredity; (2) major risk factors that can be changed — cigarette smoking, high blood pressure, elevated serum cholesterol, and physical inactivity; and (3) other contributing factors — obesity, diabetes, and stress.

MAJOR RISK FACTORS THAT CANNOT BE CHANGED

Age

The statistical probability that death will occur from heart disease increases with advancing age. All forms of cardiovascular disease contribute to the death rate (mortality), but coronary heart disease is responsible for the majority of these.[2] Nonpharmocological (no medicines) approaches that focus on exercise, proper nutrition, abstaine from tobacco, and other health promoting lifestyle behaviors contribute substantially to lowering the risk at any stage of life.

Male Gender

Men are, and have been, the primary candidates for heart disease. However, an alarming trend has surfaced in recent years. Morbidity (the sick rate in a population) and mortality (the death rate in a population) have been steadily increasing in premenopausal women. The prime contributor is cigarette smoking but when it is coupled with taking oral contraceptives, the risk increases substantially.

Coronary heart disease is the leading cause of death and disability among women, accounting for almost 250,000 deaths annually.[3] Normally, premenopausal women are unlikely candidates for heart disease unless there is a family history plus one or more of the other risk factors. Prior to menopause (permanent stoppage of the menstrual cycle) women are at less risk than men because estrogen, the female sex hormone, protects the coronary arteries from premature disease. Secondly, women have a more favorable blood fat ratio that protects the arteries from atherosclerosis. Vulnerability to heart disease for women increases after menopause because estrogen production decreases and then stops, and blood fat ratios change so that they resemble the masculine profile. By her late seventies a woman's risk is comparable to that of a man of the same age.

Heredity

Children whose parents have heart disease or atherosclerosis will have an increased tendency to develop these problems themselves. A family history of heart disease is confirmed when, (1) a father or first degree male relatives (grandfather or brothers) has had a clinically diagnosed heart attack or dies of heart disease prior to the age of 55, and (2) a mother or first degree female relatives (grandmother or sisters) has had a clinically diagnosed heart attack or dies of heart disease prior to the age of 65.[4]

MAJOR RISK FACTORS THAT CAN BE CHANGED

Cigarette Smoking

Many medical researchers consider cigarette smoking to be the most potent of the preventable risk factors associated with chronic illness and premature death. It is directly responsible for 21% of all mortality from heart disease,[5] and 35% of all cancer mortality.[6]

In the decade of the sixties, 50% of the adult males in the U.S. were smokers. Today, only 30% are smokers.[4] But smoking among women declined little if any during this time. Thirty percent of American women continue to smoke. Smoking is responsible for almost half of all heart attacks that occur to women prior to the age of 55. Rather than quit, many women have elected to switch to low yield cigarettes (low in tars and nicotine) in an effort to reduce the risk. The evidence indicates that this practice does not materially affect the risk.[7]

According to federal government statistics, smoking is rising among teenagers of both sexes. Estimates indicate that there are 3000 new teenage smokers everyday. Currently, 22% of white teenagers smoke, while 4% of African American teenagers smoke.

Harmful Products in Cigarette Smoke

Nicotine, poisonous gasses such as carbon monoxide, tars, and chemical additives to enhance flavor and taste are the harmful elements in cigarette smoke. Nicotine is a powerful addictive stimulant that has profound effects on the cardiovascular system. It contributes to spasms of the coronary blood vessels, increases the oxygen requirement of the heart at rest and during physical exertion, constricts small blood vessels so that there is a rise in blood pressure, and stimulates irregular heart beats.

Carbon monoxide is a noxious gas that is a by-product of the combustion of tobacco products. It displaces oxygen in the blood stream because hemoglobin (a protein pigment of red cells that attaches to and carries oxygen) has a much greater affinity for carbon monoxide than oxygen. As a result, the reduced oxygen carrying capacity of the blood is partially responsible for the shortness of breath that smokers experience on mild physical exertion.

The effects of cigarette smoking are insidious. Some effects occur immediately while others take years to appear. The medical profession measures the danger associated with cigarette smoking in pack years. Pack years are determined by the number of packs smoked per day multiplied by the number of years smoked. For example, smoking one pack per day for 25 years would equal 25 pack years. Smoking 1½ packs per day for 25 years would equal 37.5 pack years. The more years accumulated the more likely that the smoker will exhibit smoking-related diseases. Twenty-five years represent a typical threshold for such diseases to manifest themselves.

The Effects of Passive Smoke and Smokeless Tobacco Products

Passive smoke (also called involuntary, second-hand, or environmental smoking) involves the passive inhalation of the smoke of others. For those who must breath second-hand smoke, the risk of premature illness and death is real. Estimates show that 53,000 non-smokers die annually because of exposure to second-hand smoke.[8] The greatest number of these, 37,000, die of cardiovascular diseases, another 4000 die of lung cancer, and the remaining 12,000 die from other forms of cancer. There is a dose-response relationship between inhaling second-hand smoke and developing smoking-related illnesses. The greater the exposure, the greater the risk. No one is immune. Children of smoking parents are more likely to experience a higher incidence of influenza, bronchitis, asthma, pneumonia, and the common cold.

Smokeless tobacco products (chews, plugs, and dips) have become more popular in recent years among high school and college males. These products are considered to be a new threat to society. Nicotine is just as addictive and just as harmful when it is delivered through the oral cavity as it is when delivered through the lungs. The threat from carbon monoxide is eliminated from smokeless tobacco because these are not combustible products. Users of smokeless tobacco trade cancer risks — less risk of lung cancer, greater risk for oral cancer. The incidence of oral cancer is 50 times higher among users than among non-users.[9]

Quitting the Habit

Smoking is an extremely difficulty habit to break. To be successful, one must overcome the addiction to nicotine, and secondly, one must sever the psychological dependence on smoking. The latter is probably more of a challenge than the former. Nicotine addiction is overcome within the first couple of weeks after quitting, but the psychological and social cues are there for years. They require re-education and changes in behavior. Situations and circumstances that acted as smoking triggers in the past must be dealt with in future encounters. Smokers often light up reflexively in the presence of certain cues. Social triggers that produce smoking behavior include a cup of coffee or an alcoholic drink, the end of a meal, while talking on the telephone, where feelings of anxiety or tension occur, at parties, and

other social gatherings. The ties between these cues and smoking behavior are difficult to break.

Complicating the desire to quit, particularly among young women, is the fear of gaining weight. Cigarette smoking is to some extent a weight control technique because it is a stimulant that increases metabolism, and secondly, it speeds food through the digestive tract decreasing the time for the absorption of calories and nutrients. Cigarette smokers as a group are about 7 pounds lighter than non smokers. But smokers tend to deposit more fat in the abdomen and upper body (android fat) which increases the risk of heart attack, stroke, diabetes, and some forms of cancer.

Ninety percent of former smokers report quitting on their own.[10] Stop-smoking approaches include professional counseling, nicotine patches, nicotine chewing gum, hypnosis, artificial cigarettes, acupuncture, and aversive conditioning. The one-year success rates for these techniques range from 10% to 40%. Exercise offers another option. When people get hooked on the exercise habit, they often disconnect from the smoking habit. Smoking is a drawback to exercise performance and it limits the health gains that can be achieved with exercise. Table 5.1 includes some of the physiological changes that occur with time when one quits smoking.

Blood Pressure

Blood pressure is recorded in millimeters of mercury (mmHg). It is the force that circulating blood exerts against the artery walls. Pressure is created as the heart contracts and pumps blood into the arteries. The smallest arteries (the arterioles) offer resistance to blood flow. If the resistance is consistently high, the pressure increases and remains high. Hypertension is the medical term for high blood pressure.

Table 5.1 Incentives to Quit: Expected Body Changes That Occur With Time When One Quits Smoking

Time	Changes
20 minutes	1. Blood pressure and heart rate drop to normal values. 2. Temperature of hands and feet return to normal.
8 hours	1. Carbon monoxide in the blood returns to normal.
24 hours	1. Risk of heart attack begins to decrease.
48 hours	1. Nerve endings regenerate. 2. The senses of taste and smell improve.
2 weeks to 3 months	1. Circulation improves. 2. Lung function improves by 30%. 3. Exercise is easier to perform.
1 to 9 months	1. Coughing and sinus congestion decrease. 2. Lungs become clearer: less mucous. 3. Less respiratory infection. 4. Energy level increases. 5. Shortness of breath not as pronounced.
1 year	1. The risk of coronary heart disease is half that of a smoker.
5 years	1. Lung cancer death rate decreases by half. 2. Stroke risk is reduced to that of a nonsmoker 5 to 15 years after quitting. 3. Risk of cancer of the mouth, throat, and esophagus is half that of a nonsmoker.
10 years	1. Lung cancer death rate is similar to that of a nonsmoker. 2. Risk of cancer of the mouth, throat, esophagus, bladder, kidney, and pancreas decreases.
15 years	1. Risk of coronary heart disease is equal to that of a nonsmoker.

Adapted from "Incentives To Quit," *Your Health Network*, 2, No.1, First Quarter, 1994, p. 4.

Hypertension has no overt symptoms. It is a silent disease that can only be detected by a blood pressure screening test. Blood pressure consists of two components, (1) the systolic pressure represents the maximum pressure of blood flow in the arteries when the heart contracts, and (2) the diastolic pressure represents the minimum pressure of blood flow in the arteries between heart beats. Blood pressure is read as the systolic over the diastolic pressure. A reading of 140/90 or greater is considered to be hypertensive. A blood pressure of 100/60 is considered to be the lowest level of normal, however, some people with lower values function normally and are free of disease. It is highly desirable to have a low normal reading. Table 5.2 classifies blood pressure from normal to hypertension.

Approximately 50 million Americans have blood pressure above 140/90. The causes of 90% to 95% of these cases is unknown. This type of hypertension is classified as "essential" which is a medical term that means "of unknown origin or cause." This type of hypertension cannot be cured but it can be treated and, usually, controlled.

Long-standing uncontrolled or poorly controlled hypertension has an adverse effect on

Table 5.2 *Standards for Classification of Blood Pressure for Adults Age 18 Years and Older*

Category	Systolic (mmHg)	Diastolic (mmHg)
Normal	< 130	< 85
High Normal	130–139	85–89
Hypertension		
Stage 1 (Mild)	140–159	90–99
Stage 2 (Moderate)	160–179	100–109
Stage 3 (Severe)	180–209	110–119
Stage 4 (Very Severe)	≥ 210	≥ 120

From National Institutes of Health, *The Fifth Report of the Joint National Committee on Detection, Evaluation and Treatment of High Blood Pressure,* U.S. Dept. of Health and Human Services: NIH Publication No. 93-1088, January, 1993.

the heart. It increases its workload so that the heart enlarges in response to the strain. Since the blood pressure is consistently high, the heart gets inadequate rest. As a result the heart's muscle fibers become over-stretched and progressively lose their ability to rebound. The end result is that the force of contraction weakens and the heart becomes an inefficient pump. If intervention strategies are not enacted early in the process, the heart will suffer irreversible damage. Hypertension also has a detrimental effect on the arteries and accelerates the atherosclerotic process.

Prevention and Treatment

Prevention techniques include maintaining optimal body weight, dietary salt restriction, adequate calcium and potassium intake, voluntary relaxation, and exercise. Treatment of hypertension includes the same strategies used in prevention with the addition of medication if lifestyle behaviors fail to normalize the blood pressure.

Salt is a combination of sodium and chloride. Salt is made up of 40% sodium while the other 60% comes from chloride. Sodium is associated with raising blood pressure and is the real culprit in salt. It does so by encouraging the body to retain fluid so that the blood plasma (the liquid portion of the blood) expands. The extra blood imposes a burden on the heart which must pump blood with more force to circulate it through the arteries.

Daily salt intake should be reduced to less than two and one-half teaspoons, and this translates into less than one teaspoon of sodium. Most of the sodium consumed in the U.S. comes from processed foods. Of the remainder, 15% comes from using the salt shaker, and another 10% occurs naturally in food.[11] Heavily laden in salt are frozen dinners, frozen pizza, processed meats (bacon, ham, hot dogs, etc.), processed American style cheese, canned or dried soups, canned meats, beans, or vegetables, tomato sauce, restaurant food, and fast foods. The U.S. Surgeon General, The National Academy of Sciences, and most health professionals urge all Americans to reduce salt intake.

The jury is still out regarding the effectiveness of voluntary relaxation techniques on long-term blood pressure control. Calcium supplementation for those who are calcium deficient and hypertensive may reduce the blood pressure of some of these candidates. The same may be said of potassium supplementation.

Aerobic exercises, such as walking and jogging, contribute to blood pressure control. Based on the evidence, The American College of Sports Medicine (ACSM) has taken the position that "endurance (aerobic) exercise training by individuals at high risk for developing hypertension will reduce the rise in blood pressure that occurs with time."[12] Furthermore, aerobic exercises performed at moderate intensity (40% to 70% of the aerobic capacity) appear to lower blood pressure as much as, and sometimes more so, than exercises performed at higher intensities.

There are several possibilities regarding the mechanisms through which aerobic exercise lowers blood pressure. First, epinephrine and norepinephrine are hormones secreted by the body that play important roles in the regulation of blood pressure. Both are vasoconstrictors, that is, they clamp down on the arterioles which then requires more force to circulate blood through them. Aerobic training decreases the circulating levels of these hormones allowing the arterioles to relax and widen. In other words, exercise keeps the arteries limber. This response lowers the resistance to blood flow which in turn lowers the blood pressure.

Second, aerobic exercise increases the cell's sensitivity to insulin. Insulin is a hormone manufactured by the body that facilitates the passage of sugar from the blood to the cells. Sugar (glucose) is an important source of energy that is used by the cells to perform their normal functions. Increased sensitivity to insulin by the cells leads to an important bonus: excess sodium is excreted by the kidneys and this also lowers the blood pressure. Third, aerobic exercise contributes to weight loss which is effective in lowering the blood pressure.

High Serum Cholesterol

Cholesterol is a steroid required for the manufacture of hormones, bile (for the digestion and absorption of fats), it is one of the structural components of neural tissue, and it is required for the construction of cell walls. A certain amount of cholesterol is needed for good health, but an excessive amount in the blood (known as serum cholesterol) is associated with heart attacks and strokes. Strokes occur when blood clots block the flow of blood to portions of the brain or when a hemorrhage occurs in the brain due to a blood vessel that has burst. Paralysis of one side of the body and slurred speech are some of the consequences that occur to victims of a stroke. If a stroke is massive, the victim will die.

We obtain cholesterol in two ways, (1) through the dietary consumption of it, and (2) the body manufactures its own. Currently males are consuming 376 milligrams (mg) of cholesterol daily and females are consuming 259 milligrams.[13] The American Heart Association (AHA) recommends daily consumption of less than 300 mg. In 1960, the dietary intake of cholesterol by males was 706 mg per day while females were consuming 493 mg per day. Americans have made significant progress in reducing dietary cholesterol in the last three decades. However, we need no dietary intake of cholesterol because the liver manufactures all of the cholesterol that the body needs. Saturated fat is the primary ingredient from which cholesterol is produced inside the body. As a result, most authorities are more concerned about the amount of saturated fat consumption rather than cholesterol consumption, but they are quick to add that it is prudent to limit the intake of both. Dietary cholesterol and saturated fat are found in animal flesh, eggs, whole milk, and whole milk dairy products. Fruits and vegetables are free of cholesterol, and with a few exceptions, are also low in fat. Coconuts, coconut oil, palm oil, and palm kernal oil are high in saturated fat. Olives, nuts and seeds, and avocados are high in monounsaturated fat which is a less harmful form. Regardless, AHA guidelines indicate that consumption should be less than 30% of the total caloric intake.

The amount of cholesterol circulating in the blood is expressed in milligrams per deciliter (mg/dL) so that a cholesterol level of 210 is read as 210 mg/dL. Table 5.3 indicates levels where blood cholesterol becomes a risk.

Table 5.3 Serum Cholesterol — Relative Risk

Cholesterol (mg/dL)	Level of Risk
< 200*	Desirable
200–239	Borderline
≥ 240**	High

  * < less than
** ≥ equal to or greater than

Reducing and maintaining a desirable value of serum cholesterol keeps the risk at a lower level. For every 1% that serum cholesterol is lowered, the risk of heart disease is reduced by 2% to 3%.[14]

The Cholesterol Carriers

Knowing one's total serum cholesterol value tells only part of the story. To fully evaluate the cholesterol risk, we must know our total cholesterol (TC) as well as two of its important fractions — the low density lipoprotein fraction (LDL) and the high density lipoprotein fraction (HDL). The lipoproteins are carriers to which cholesterol attaches for transport through the circulatory system.

The most atherogenic (capable of producing atherosclerosis) of the carriers is the low density lipoprotein group (LDL). This fraction is the primary transporter of cholesterol from the liver to the cells of the body. The liver and cells have receptor sites that lock-on to the LDLs so that their cargo of cholesterol and other fats can be assimilated for use by them. Under normal conditions, the cells effectively remove cholesterol from circulation, but when LDL concentrations are excessive, the receptor sites become saturated impeding further removal. The net result is a rise in blood concentrations of both LDL and cholesterol. The excess LDLs are oxidized in the cells of the artery walls. This is the beginning of atherosclerosis and the formation of plaques that eventually clog the arteries supplying blood to the heart or brain. The LDL concentration may be lowered through weight loss, and reduction in the intake of saturated fat, total fat, and cholesterol. Table 5.4 presents the relative risk associated with LDL cholesterol.

Table 5.4 Guidelines for LDL Cholesterol Risk

LDL Cholesterol (mg/dL)	Risk
< 130*	Desirable
130–159	Borderline-High
> 160**	High

  * < less than
** > greater than

A second, very important cholesterol carrier is the high density lipoprotein (HDL) fraction. The HDLs are involved in reverse transport, that is, they scavenge cholesterol from the tissues and blood stream and transfer it back to the liver through intermediary carriers for degradation, recycling, or disposal. HDLs protect the arteries from atherosclerosis by clearing cholesterol from the blood. The higher the HDL count, the better. A low number of circulating HDLs is a powerful independent predictor of heart disease. Table 5.5 presents HDL values and their relative degree of risk.

Table 5.5 HDL Values and Degree of Relative Risk by Gender

HDL Cholesterol (mg/dL)	Risk
45	Average for males
55	Average for females
< 25	Triple the risk for males
< 40*	Triple the risk for females

* < less than

Table 5.6 Ratio of Total Cholesterol to HDL

Risk	Male	Female
Very Low (1/2 of average)	< 3.4*	< 3.3
Low	4.0	3.8
Average	5.0	4.5
Moderate (2 × average)	9.5	7.0
High (3 × average)	> 23**	> 11.0

* < less than
** > greater than

HDLs may be increased through aerobic exercise, weight loss, and moderate alcohol intake. Moderate intake refers to approximately one ounce of alcohol per day for males and one-half ounce for females. Approximately one-half to two-thirds of an ounce is found in 12 ounces of beer, 5 ounces of wine, and 1.5 ounces of 80 proof spirits. You should be very careful regarding alcohol intake. It is rich in calories, second only to fat. Avoid alcohol if you are watching your weight, if you intend to drive, or if there are alcoholic tendencies in your family.

Determining the Cholesterol Risk

An accurate assessment of the cholesterol risk requires the measurement of total cholesterol (TC) and the LDL and HDL fractions. A desirable total cholesterol can still be a significant risk if the LDLs are too high or the HDLs are too low. Another clue regarding risk is provided by the ratio between total cholesterol and HDL. Dividing total cholesterol by HDL yields an index number that is interpreted with the aid of Table 5.6.

Physical Inactivity

Physical inactivity is debilitating to the human body. Humans are exponents of the biological dictate "use it, or lose it." That which we use becomes stronger while that which we do not use becomes weaker. All body systems and all muscles, including the heart muscle, respond to this principle.

The results of a number of recently completed, important investigations, concluded that physical inactivity is major risk for heart disease. Those who exercise consistently, even at low intensity, tend to be healthier and to live longer than people who are sedentary. The ongoing Harvard Alumni Study found that the minimum exercise threshold for increasing longevity was as little as walking five miles per week.[15] Optimal benefits were achieved by those who walked or jogged 20 to 22 miles per week. They lived on the average two years longer than sedentary people. Investigators at the Dallas Aerobics Center found that physically fit subjects who had high blood pressure or elevated serum cholesterol were less likely to die prematurely from all causes than unfit individuals with normal values of both.[16] The Centers for Disease Control concluded that exercise is the one lifestyle change that could most affect the health status of this nation.[17] This is based primarily on the fact that 80% of Americans are either sedentary or exercise too infrequently to enhance their health.

Health enhancement through physical activity does not require a great deal of effort. The requirement is 30 minutes of physical activity at least four days per week every week. There are few constraints on the type of activities that can be chosen. All physical activities (cycling, jogging, walking, swimming, etc), most games and sports, many leisure time activities, and some occupational work has the potential to meet the minimum criteria for improving your health. A summary of selected health benefits appears in Table 5.7.

Exercise on a regular basis has been emphasized in this text because it is the only way to improve fitness and health status simultaneously. There is another very important reason for stressing consistent participation. The risk of sudden death from a heart attack during and immediately after physical exertion rises dramatically for those who are not fit or who exercise sporadically. Two recent studies, one completed in the United States and the other in Germany, documented this observation. The U.S. study showed that sedentary people were 100 times more vulnerable to suffering a heart attack during strenuous activity than at other times.[18] In contrast, those who exercise consistently face only a small increase in the risk but the health and fitness benefits that are achieved from training far outweigh the minimal risk.[19]

Table 5.7 *Summary of Selected Health Benefits from Aerobic Exercise*

I.   Reduces the risk of cardiovascular disease
   1. Increase HDL-cholesterol
   2. Decreases LDL-cholesterol
   3. Favorably changes the ratios between total cholesterol and HDL-C, and between LDL-C and HDL-cholesterol
   4. Decreases triglyceride levels
   5. Promotes relaxation; relieves stress and tension
   6. Decreases body fat and favorably changes body composition
   7. Reduces blood pressure especially if it is high
   8. Blood platelets are less sticky
   9. Less cardiac arrhythmias
   10. Increases myocardial efficiency
      a. Lowers resting heart rate
      b. Increases stroke volume
   11. Increases oxygen-carrying capacity of the blood

II.   Helps control diabetes
   1. Cells are less resistant to insulin
   2. Reduces body fat

III. Develops stronger bones that are less susceptible to injury

IV.   Promotes joint stability by
   1. Increasing muscular strength
   2. Increasing strength of the ligaments, tendons, cartilage, and connective tissues

V.   Contributes to fewer low back problems

VI.   Acts as a stimulus for other lifestyle changes

VII. Improves self-concept

OTHER CONTRIBUTING FACTORS

Obesity

The current perception of obesity is that it is a chronic disease like hypertension or diabetes rather than a simple failure of willpower.[20] Data collected from 1988 to 1991 indicated that Americans are once again gaining weight. During this time period, the number of overweight males rose from 24% to 32% while the number of overweight females rose from 27% to 35%.

Excess body weight carries medical consequences. Obesity is not only a disease but it increases the risk and the consequences of many other chronic diseases. It significantly increases the workload of the heart, and it coexists with high blood pressure and elevated serum cholesterol. Obesity is related to the onset of diabetes, arthritis, and some forms of cancer.

Obesity is defined by the National Institute of Health as 20% above desirable weight. Other authorities define it relative to the percent of body weight that consists of fat. This is a more accurate method that provides guidelines for weight loss and weight control. Males are obese when 23% to 25% or more of their total body weight is in the form of fat. Females are obese when 32% or more of their total body weight is in the form of fat.

Excessive fat is a risk but the manner in which it is distributed must also be considered. Abdominal fat — also known as "android," "central," or "masculine pattern" fat — increases the risk for heart attacks, stroke, diabetes, and some forms of cancer. Even as few as 15 extra pounds stored in this pattern substantially increases the risk. Fat that is stored in the hips, buttocks, and thighs — also known as

"gynoid" fat or "feminine pattern" fat — presents less of a risk.

Fortunately obesity is reversible. When the excess weight is lost, the risk subsides. Weight loss strategies will be discussed in Chapter 7.

Diabetes Mellitus

Diabetes mellitus is a metabolic disorder in which the body is unable to regulate the level of blood glucose (sugar). It is one of the 10 leading causes of death in the U.S. Diabetics who die prematurely succumb to the complications of the disease. These include cardiovascular lesions, accelerated atherosclerosis, and heart disease. Diabetics are also susceptible to kidney disease, nerve and blood vessel damage, blindness, and lower limb amputation resulting from gangrene. In addition, diabetes tends to elevate serum cholesterol and creates an environment in the circulatory system that facilitates the development of blood clots. Many physicians are convinced that diabetes is a major risk for coronary heart disease.[21]

There are two types of diabetes mellitus. Type I usually occurs early in life. Victims of Type I diabetes don't produce insulin so they must take it by daily injection. Insulin is a hormone that regulates blood sugar by moving it, when appropriate, from the blood to the cells where it can be used to fuel the cell's needs. Without insulin, sugar would accumulate in the blood and spill out of the body through the kidneys. The body would be forced to use fat as its primary fuel and this produces serious consequences for the diabetic. Diabetes cannot be cured, but it can be controlled. Living a well-regulated life that includes exercise, weight control, and a low fat diet are paramount to the control of Type I diabetes.

Type II diabetes occurs about middle age to overweight, underactive people. This form of diabetes may or may not require medication.

Lifestyle factors are important in the treatment and control of Type II diabetes. Exercise and weight loss combine to increase cellular sensitivity to insulin so that blood sugar can be normalized with less insulin. Each bout of exercise reduces blood platelet adhesiveness for about 24 hours. This lessens the advent of a heart attack by decreasing the likelihood of a coronary spasm. Many physicians encourage their diabetic patients to walk as the preferred form of exercise.

A landmark piece of research, The Physician's Health Study, was a large scale collaborative effort that showed that exercise reduced the risk of developing Type II diabetes.[22] Type II accounts for 90% of all cases of diabetes that occur in middle age. Physicians who exercised vigorously five or more times per week had a 42% reduction in the incidence of Type II diabetes compared to those who exercised less than one time per week. The reduction in the risk was particularly evident among those at greatest risk — the obese. The researchers concluded that at least 24% of all Type II diabetes was related to a sedentary lifestyle.

Stress

Stress is difficult to quantify. However, authorities tend to agree that chronic stress or distress produces physiological changes in the body that may predispose people to illness. Secondly, it may hasten the process of subclinical disease (latent disease — not yet detectable).

The immune system may be detrimentally affected for months or years as the result of chronic stress. Chronic stress stimulates the secretion of above normal amounts of hormones (collectively called the catecholamines) that circulate at high levels in the blood stream. The catecholamines rev up the body's engine so that it runs at high throttle. Physical exercise is the antidote because it metabolizes these products thereby lowering their level in the blood. But, the catecholamine level of sedentary people remains elevated so that the arterioles (the smallest arteries) are in a constant state of slight contraction. This condition, known as peripheral vascular resistance, increases the workload of the heart. A review of the scientific literature indicates that aerobic exercise reduces peripheral vascular resistance, decreases the severity of the stress response, shortens the recovery time from stress, and reduces stress-related vulnerability to disease.

Situations and circumstances are stressful only if we allow them to be. It is not the stressor that produces the problem, it is the way we perceive and react to it. Two people confronted by the same stressor might exhibit different reactions. For example, delivering a speech to a group of people may be anxiety producing and threatening for one of them while it may be accepted as an exciting challenge to another. We cannot avoid stress, it is part of life in a competitive dynamic society such as our own. We are currently entering the age of information. This will exert rapid changes in our educational and occupational lives. The information super highway will compound the normal stressful life change events that occur to many of us. Divorce, death of a loved one, furloughed from one's job, retirement, etc., are stressful events that must be dealt with. Since we cannot avoid stress, we must learn to manage it. Exercise is a great coping mechanism that rids the body of stress-initiated harmful products that accumulate over time.

Summary

- The leading form of cardiovascular disease claiming nearly 500,000 lives annually is coronary heart disease.

- Coronary heart disease is characterized by obstructions (blood clots or spasms) that occur to the coronary arteries that lead to a reduction or stoppage of blood flow to portions of the heart muscle.

- Atherosclerosis is a slow progressive disease of large and mid-size arteries.

- Risk factors are genetic or learned behaviors that increase the probability of premature illness and death from a specific chronic disease.

- The statistical probability that death will occur from heart disease increases with advancing age.

- Children whose parents have heart disease or atherosclerosis will have a increased tendency to develop these problems.

- Cigarette smoking is responsible for 21% of all mortality from heart disease.

- Smoking is rising among teenagers of both sexes.

- Nicotine is a powerful addictive stimulant that has profound adverse effect on the cardiovascular system.

- Carbon monoxide displaces oxygen and reduces the oxygen carrying capacity of the blood.

- The danger of cigarette smoking is measured in pack years.

- Breathing smoke is harmful to nonsmokers.

- Smokeless tobacco products are addictive and harmful.

- Many cigarette smokers, particularly women, won't quit for fear of gaining weight.

- Hypertension is the medical term for high blood pressure.

- Essential hypertension is the most common form of high blood pressure.

- Lifestyle behaviors that may prevent or treat hypertension include exercise, weight loss, salt restriction, calcium and potassium intake, and voluntary relaxation techniques.

- The consumption of cholesterol in the U.S. has been decreasing since 1960.

- Cholesterol is found in animal flesh, eggs, whole milk, and whole milk dairy products.

- The liver manufactures cholesterol from saturated fat so it is important to reduce our intake of this form of fat.

- LDL cholesterol is implicated in the development of atherosclerosis.

- HDL cholesterol protects the arteries by removing cholesterol from the blood.

- Those who exercise consistently tend to be healthier and live longer than people who are sedentary.

- Thirty minutes of physical activity most days of the week is currently recommended for health enhancement.

- The risk of sudden death during and immediately after exercise is much more likely to occur to unfit people.

- The number of overweight people increased from 1988 to 1991.

- Obesity is a disease and a risk factor for other chronic diseases.

▶ The android pattern of fat deposition increases the risk of heart disease, stroke, diabetes, and some forms of cancer.

▶ Diabetes mellitus is a metabolic disorder in which the body is unable to regulate the level of blood glucose.

▶ Type I diabetes usually occurs early in life and requires the daily injection of insulin.

▶ Type II diabetes usually occurs about middle-age to overweight and underexercised people.

▶ The Physician's Health Study concluded that a least 24% of all Type II diabetes is related to a sedentary lifestyle.

▶ Stress suppresses the immune system.

▶ Since we cannot avoid stress, we must learn to manage it.

▶ REFERENCES

1. American Heart Association, *Heart and Stroke Facts: 1994 Statistical Supplement*, Dallas: American Heart Association, 1994.

2. Van Camp, S. P., and Boyer, J. L. "Cardiovascular Aspects of Aging," *Physician and Sportsmedicine* 17, No. 4: (1989), p. 121.

3. Bush, T. L. "Influence On Cholesterol and Lipoprotein Levels In Women," *Cholesterol and Coronary Disease — Reducing Risk*, 2, No. 6: (1990), p. 1.

4. Grundy, S. "Decline in Coronary Heart Disease Mortality: Primary Factors and Secondary Interventions," *Cholesterol and Coronary Disease — Reducing the Risk*, 4, No. 4: (1993), p. 1.

5. Manson, J. E. et al. "The Primary Prevention of Myocardial Infraction," *New England Journal of Medicine* 326, No. 21: (1992), p. 1406.

6. *Cancer Facts and Figures — 1994*, Atlanta, GA: American Cancer Society, 1994.

7. Grundy, S.

8. Palmer, J. R. et al. "Low Yield Cigarettes and the Risk of Nonfatal Myocardial Infarction in Women," *New England Journal of Medicine*, 320, No. 21: (1989), p. 1569.

9. "Passive Smoking: A Threat to Health?", *Harvard Health Letter*, 3: (1991), p.. 8.

10. Department of Health and Human Services. *Reducing the Health Consequences of Smoking: 25 Years of Progress: A Report of the Surgeon General*, Washington, DC: U.S. Government Printing Office, 1989. DHHS Publication Number (CDC), 89-8411.

11. Liebman, B. "The Salt Shakeout," *Nutrition Action Health Letter*, 21, No. 2: (March, 1994), p. 5.

12. American College of Sports Medicine. "Physical Activity, Physical Fitness, and Hypertension," *Medicine and Science in Sports and Exercise*, 25, No. 10: (1993), p. i.

13. "Fascinating Facts." *University of California at Berkeley Wellness Letter* 10, Issue 6: (March, 1994), p. 1.

14. La Rosa, J. C. et al. "The Cholesterol Facts: A Summary of the Evidence Relating Dietary Fats, Serum Cholesterol, and Coronary Heart Disease: A Joint Statement by the American Heart Association and the National Heart Lung, and Blood Institute," *Circulation*, 81: (1990), p. 1721.

15. Paffenbarger, R. S. et al. "Physical Activity, All Cause Mortality, and Longevity of College Alumni," *New England Journal of Medicine*, 314: (1986), p. 253.

16. Blair, S. N. et al. "Physical Fitness and All-Cause Mortality — A Prospective Study of Healthy Men and Women, *Journal of the American Medical Association*, 262: (1989), p. 2395.

17. Powell, K. E., et al. "Physical Activity and the Incidence of Coronary Heart Disease," *Annual Review of Public Health*, 8: (1987), p. 253.

18. Mittleman, M. A. et al. "Triggering of Acute Myocardial Infarction By Heavy Physical Exertion" *The New England Journal of Medicine*, 329: (1993), p. 1677.

19. Willich, S. N. et al. "Physical Exertion As A Trigger Of Acute Myocardial Infarction," *The New England Journal of Medicine*, 329: (1993), p. 1684.

20. "Losing Weight: A New Attitude Emerges." *Harvard Heart Letter*, 4, No. 7: (March, 1994), p. 1.

21. Grundy, S.

22. Manson, J. E. et al. "A Prospective Study of Exercise and Incidence of Diabetes Among U.S. Male Physicians," *Journal of the American Medical Association* 268: (1992), p. 268.

Reducing the Risk of Chronic Diseases: The Role of Exercise

This chapter focuses on cancer, osteoporosis, osteo-arthritis, asthma, and stress. These chronic diseases were selected because of their prevalence in the United States and because a relationship exists between them and exercise. Exercising regularly has a modifying or preventive effect on each of them.

CANCER

Cancer, the second leading cause of death in the U.S., is responsible for one in every five deaths.[1] Projected estimates for 1994 indicate that 538,000 people will die from cancer and 1,208,000 new cases will be diagnosed. The incidence of cancer has been on the increase during the last 50 years. This is due to the rise in the number of cases of lung cancer. If lung cancer deaths were excluded, cancer mortality would have declined by 14% during this period of time.

Cancer is a general term that applies to more than 100 diseases that are characterized by abnormal and uncontrolled cellular growth. Any cell can become cancerous if it is exposed under the right conditions to carcinogenic (cancer-producing) substances. Exposure to carcinogens will eventually cause mutant cells that divide and grow uncontrollably.

Normal cells follow an orderly and predictable blue-print for growth and division. In adulthood this is restricted to the replacement of lost cells. Cancerous cells do not respond to the body's signals restricting cellular division so that they and their offspring continue to grow wildly. The mass of new growth is a tumor or neoplasm (new tissue). Cancerous tumors are malignant, they grow rapidly, and they are not confined or localized. They shed their cells, invade surrounding tissues, and compete with normal cells for space and nutrients. Metastasis is the medical term for the spread of cancer from its original site to other areas of the body.

The processes that transform normal cells to malignant ones are complex and not well understood. Normal genes that undergo mutation may become oncogenes or cancerous genes. When oncogenes divide, they pass on their malignant characteristics to their progeny. Scientists are attempting to identify the products manufactured and given off by oncogenes. If these are distinguishable, they can be used as markers to detect cancer in its very early and most treatable stage.

The Strategies of Prevention

Techniques and strategies have emerged that can reduce the incidence of many forms of cancer. Cancer prevention includes: (1) abstinence from all forms of tobacco, (2) a diet rich in fruits, vegetables, and grains, that is low in fat, and devoid of smoked and cured meat and fish, (3) minimum exposure to radiation and carcinogenic chemicals, and (4) regular exercise participation.

Exercise diminishes the risk of colon cancer, breast cancer, and may slow the progression of other malignancies as well.[2] At least eight groups of research teams have investigated the relationship between exercise and colon cancer since 1980. Seven of them concluded that exercise lowers the risk and that leading a sedentary life increases the risk by 50%. It doesn't take much exercise to achieve the protection. Expending 1000 calories per week in physical activity — the equivalent of walking or jogging 10 miles a week — cuts the risk of colon cancer nearly in half.[3]

More than 5000 middle-aged women were grouped according to their participation in college varsity or intramural sports during their early adult lives.[4] The researchers assumed that former athletes would be more active later in life than those who were sedentary as young adults. The two groups were compared for the onset of cancer of the breast and reproductive system. The differences between the two groups were dramatic — the nonathletic group had 86% more breast cancer than the athletic group and they were 153% more likely to develop cancers of the reproductive system.

How Exercise Works to Prevent Cancer

At present, the mechanisms through which exercise contributes to the prevention of cancer are speculative, but plausible. Regarding its effect on colon cancer, the most accepted of the theories is the rapid-transit hypothesis. Physical activity promotes bowel movements. This reduces the contact time that potentially carcinogenic substances in fecal matter have with the intestinal walls. Reduced contact time means reduced risk.

The leading theory regarding the effect of physical activity on breast cancer is that the amount of body fat is lower in active women. Stored fat drives the production of the female sex hormone estrogen which is implicated in the development of cancers of the reproductive system. A reduction in stored fat lessens the drive, reduces the production of estrogen and decreases stimulation to cells with malignant potential. Reduction of body fat in males lessens the overall cancer risk.

In addition to lowering the fat content of the body, exercise stimulates the immune system by increasing the production of cancer fighting chemicals and enhancing the killing power of certain cells. Moderate amounts of exercise at moderate intensity seem to promote these functions best, while prolonged, very vigorous exercise may depress the effectiveness of the immune system. Highly trained endurance-type competitive athletes often report an increase in the common cold, flu, and upper respiratory infections during heavy training and after competition. This is an indicator of a weakened immune system.[5] While very heavy exercise may depress the immune system, the problem for most people in the U.S. is too little exercise rather than too much.

OSTEOPOROSIS

Osteoporosis literally means porous bone. It is a "silent condition" characterized by the gradual loss of bone mass. As a result the bones become brittle and vulnerable to fracturing as we age. Two types of osteoporosis have been identified. Type I affects eight times more women than men and occurs after menopause. The process accelerates at about age 50 when estrogen production begins to decline. The major sites of fracture in order of frequency are compression fractures of the vertebrae of the spine followed by fractures of the wrist. Type I osteoporosis is a major cause of disability among older women.[6]

Type II osteoporosis affects twice as many women as men and occurs to both sexes at approximately 70 years of age.[7] Hip fractures are the most frequent events and estrogen deficiency is only one of many possible contributing factors.

The Risk Factors For Osteoporosis

Some of the factors that increase the likelihood of developing osteoporosis are:

Age: Osteoporosis takes many years to develop so that the longer one lives the greater the probability of developing this disease.

Gender: Women are more susceptible than men particularly those with small, thin skeletal framework or those who experience early menopause. Hormone replacement therapy (HRT) during and after menopause may be necessary. The decision to take HRT should be based on risk versus benefit and it should be made by patient and physician together.

Heredity: The offspring of parents who have osteoporosis are at greater risk.

Lack of Physical Activity: Weight bearing exercises and resistance exercises increase the strength and thickness of bones. Conversely, lack of stimulation from sedentary living contributes to the loss of bone minerals.

Cigarette Smoking: Cigarette smoking suppresses estrogen levels and leads to premature menopause so that bone loss occurs earlier in life.

Insufficient Calcium Intake: Sufficient dietary intake of calcium is necessary for the development and maintenance of strong bones. The recommended daily intake of calcium is 800 milligrams (mg) but adolescents, young adults, and pregnant or lactating women require 1200 mg a day. Post-menopausal women should consume from 1200 10 1500 mg per day.

Osteoporosis is treatable but it is not curable. The best approach is to prevent or delay its advent. The most important preventive technique is to develop as much bone as possible during the teenage years. About 45% of an individual's bone mass is formed during this time.[8] To achieve this increase involves a sufficient intake of calcium and a regular program of weight bearing and resistance type exercise. Unfortunately, most female teenagers do neither, therefore, setting themselves up for skeletal problems later in life.

The Effects of Exercise

Bone is living tissue that responds to the downward force of gravity and the lateral forces generated by the forceful contraction of muscles. Weight bearing, impact loading exercises such as walking, jogging, aerobic dancing, and stair climbing can increase bone mass.[9] Even the skeletal systems of nursing home residents (average age 81 years) have responded to exercise with an increase in bone mass. Non-weight-bearing activities such as swimming and stationary cycling are not as effective in increasing bone density.[10]

Researchers have examined the effect of resistance weight training on the skeletal system. Studies have indicated that bones respond to weight training by becoming thicker and denser.[11] For good results, weight training exercises should be performed at an intensity level equal to 85% of one repetition maximum (1RM). This is approximately equivalent to performing 10 lifts, or repetitions, of an exercise with a weight that cannot be lifted 11 times. Exercises should be selected that stress the major muscle groups so that the bones they are attached to will also be stressed.

▶ OSTEOARTHRITIS

Osteoarthritis is the most common of the many forms of arthritis. Osteoarthritis leads to the decline of the soft, smooth cartilage at the surface of joints. This occurs to some people as early as 30 years of age.

There are two types of osteoarthritis: primary and secondary. Primary osteoarthritis is the result of normal use and is referred to as "wear and tear" arthritis. The joints most commonly affected are the thumb and end joints of the other fingers, the hips, knees, neck, and lower spine.[12] Secondary osteoarthritis may occur from one or a combination of the following: (1) joint injury, (2) disease, and, (3) chronic traumas imposed by obesity, poor posture, and occupational overuse. Osteoarthritis causes minimal inflammation of the affected joints.

One of the myths that seems to persist is that jogging causes premature osteoarthritis of the knees. This perception is fueled by the biomechanics of jogging which indicates that the force developed at the knee when the foot strikes the ground is six times that of the force generated by walking. As a result, many have concluded that jogging must be harmful to the knees. However, 35 years of data collected by researchers in the Framingham Heart Study indicated that the major cause of osteoarthritis of the knees is obesity.[13] In fact, high mileage running — an average of 28 miles per week for a minimum of 12 years — was not associated with the premature development of osteoarthritis.

Osteoarthritics need to exercise because it increases strength, promotes flexibility, reduces pain, controls body weight, preserves mobility, and enhances well being. The health of cartilage, which has no blood supply of its own, depends on regular stimulation and use of the joints. When the joints move, fluid and waste products are squeezed out of cartilage. When the joint relaxes, fluid seeps back in, bringing oxygen and nutrients with it. Rhythmic contractions of the muscles lubricate and nourish the joints.

If osteoarthritis is already present, impact loading exercises may aggravate the condition and produce pain. If this occurs, a simple shift to low impact nonweight-bearing exercises should bring relief and allow continued participation. Appropriate activities include walking, water walking, water aerobics and swimming. Other acceptable activities include the use of stationary cycles, rowing machines, and cross-country ski machines.

ASTHMA

The American Thoracic Society defines asthma as the increased responsiveness of the trachea (wind pipe) and bronchi (the two main subdivisions of the trachea that transport air to and from the lungs) to a variety of stimuli resulting in airway obstruction that is reversible spontaneously or as a result of treatment. Breathing becomes very difficult during an asthma attack and this can be a frightening experience.

Nine million Americans are asthmatic and there are approximately 5000 asthma-related deaths each year in the U.S.[14] Asthma affects 5% to 10% of all Americans age 5 to 21 years.[15] There is no cure for asthma but there are medications that effectively prevent or reduce the length and severity of an attack.

There are many potential triggering mechanisms that can provoke an asthma attack. These include cold dry air, exercise, viral infections, emotions, sinus infection, and environmental irritants. Substances and conditions such as these, that precipitate an asthma attack in some people while producing no abnormal reactions in others are termed allergens.

The fear of exercise-induced asthma (EIA) is the reason that many asthmatics remain sedentary. But asthma should not be a deterrent to participating in physical activities by children, adolescents, or older adults. The American Academy of Allergy and Immunology encourages regular exercise for asthmatics because they receive the same health benefits as other individuals. Asthma suffers have competed in sports at the national and international levels. In 1984, 11% of the U.S. Olympic Team consisted of athletes who had asthma or exercise-induced asthma.[16] Collectively, these asthmatic athletes, 67 of them, won 41 Olympic medals. Their success was due to the combination of medical preventive treatment and their high level of physical fitness.

Asthmatics who want to exercise or who are currently exercising can use the same method of prevention practiced by the Olympic athletes. First, airway-opening drugs should be used immediately prior to exercise or competition. Second, a gradual warm-up period of 15 minutes should be followed by a 15 minute period of rest. This protocol reduces the probability of incurring exercise-induced asthma for about two hours. Third, treatment must be individualized to find the optimal regimen for each individual. This will involve several trial and error attempts before the best approach is found. Turn your attention to Table 6.1 for a more complete set of exercise guidelines.

The types and intensity of exercise that contribute to the onset of exercise-induced asthma have been identified. The mechanisms responsible for EIA are the loss of respiratory heat and water due to the high rate of breathing during exercise. The more intense the exercise the greater the loss of heat and water, therefore the more intense forms of exercise are generally the most asthmogenic (capable of inducing bronchospasms). Swimming and other water activities are the least asthmogenic types of exercise. This is probably due to the warm, moist environment in which they are performed and secondly, because the high breathing rates required to precipitate bronchospasms are difficult to achieve.[17] Running and cycling appear to be the most asthmogenic of the outdoor activities but the risk can be minimized by following the guidelines in Table 6.1.

▶ STRESS

Stress is the nonspecific response of the human organism to any demand, positive or negative, that it encounters. Stress results from any event, condition, or situation that creates change, threat, or loss. These events are referred to as stressors or "stress triggers." Events, conditions, and circumstances have stress-producing potential but their effect on a given individual depends on the individual's response. When stressors appear to overload or exceed one's ability to cope, the results can be harmful and the consequences are proportional to the response.

The reaction to a stressor determines its power to induce stress. For example, having to make a speech to a group of people might be a stressor of crisis proportions for one person, while the same event might be an exciting challenge to another.

We cannot avoid stress. Even if we moved to a remote mountain hideaway or an uninhabited island we still could not avoid stress because this type of existence would have its own set of stressful circumstances. Since stress cannot be avoided, the healthy alternative is that we must learn to manage it. There is a short verse, The Serenity Prayer, that is extremely wise in its philosophy and guiding principles. If we apply it, life's tribulations will be placed in proper context and therefore easier to manage. It states: "God, grant me the serenity to accept things I cannot change, courage to change the things I can, and wisdom to know the difference." It may take a lifetime to behave in a manner consistent with the principles of this prayer. The earlier we begin, the more gracefully we can cope with the stressful changes in our lives.

Researchers indicate that too many changes, bad or good, occurring within a one-year

---

▶ Table 6.1   Guidelines for Exercise for Asthmatics

Asthmatics can benefit from exercise. Swimming and other water activities are best, but other forms of exercise can be beneficial when guidelines are followed:

▶ Take medications as prescribed by your physician.

▶ Perform a 5 to 10 minute warm-up that includes moderate stretching.

▶ Gradually increase the pace during the first 10 to 15 minutes of exercise, being careful to keep the heart rate below 140 beats per minute.

▶ As your physical tolerance to exercise increases, you can gradually increase the intensity and/or duration of exercise.

▶ Breathe slowly through your nose as much as possible because nasal breathing reduces the likelihood of hyperventilation and humidifies and warms the air before it enters the lungs.

▶ Breathe through a scarf or mask if you exercise outdoors during the winter.

▶ Avoid exposure to allergens and air pollutants by exercising indoors during air pollution alerts. Exercise in areas with minimal auto traffic (public parks, golf courses).

▶ Recognize that the pollen count is highest in the early morning hours.

▶ Do a gradual cooldown to avoid rapid thermal changes in the airways.

Adapted from Rosato, F., *Fitness For Wellness — The Physical Connection*, St. Paul: West Publishing CO., 1994.

period of time increases the probability of a health-related problem soon after. Table 6.2 presents the Life Events Scale — Student Version that reflects the potential effects of 31 stressors from those requiring the greatest personal adjustment to those requiring the least. Death of a loved one, divorce between parents, and being fired from a job are significantly stressful events. Note that positive life changes, such as marriage and pregnancy, are also stress-inducing. The former are negative stressors (distressors) while the latter are positive stressors (eustressors). It is important to understand that the predictability of life event scales is limited. While they identify stressors, the individual's response to a stressful event, rather than the event itself, determines its impact. Read the directions for using Table 6.2 and complete the exercise.

Directions — Life Events Scale

Table 6.2 is an adaptation of the Homes-Rahe Life Events Scale. This scale focuses on those events that typically affect college-age people. Respond to the changes in your life by checking those items that you have experienced during the past year. Total the points and interpret the results as follows:

1. **300 points or more** — high risk of developing a health problem or experiencing a negative health change in the following year.

2. **150–300 points** — you have a 50-50 chance of experiencing a negative health change within two years.

3. **Less than 150 points** — you have a one-in-three chance of experiencing a negative health change in the next couple of years.

Note: Remember, it is your reaction to life changes rather than the change itself that produces the seriousness of the stress. Deal

Table 6.2 Life Events Scale — Student Version

EVENT	LIFE CHANGE UNITS
Death of close family member	100
Death of a close friend	73
Divorce between parents	65
Jail term	63
Major personal injury or illness	63
Marriage	58
Fired from job	50
Failed important course	47
Change in health of family member	45
Pregnancy	45
Sex problems	44
Serious argument with close friend	40
Change in financial status	39
Trouble with parents	39
Change in major	39
New girlfriend or boyfriend	38
Increased workload at school	37
Outstanding personal achievement	36
First quarter/semester in college	35
Change in living conditions	31
Serious argument with instructor	30
Lower grades than expected	29
Change in sleeping habits	29
Change in social activities	29
Change in eating habits	28
Chronic car trouble	26
Change in number of family get togethers	26
Too many missed classes	25
Change of college/change of work	24
Dropped more than one class	23
Minor traffic violations	20

Your Score   _____

How do you interpret your score?   _____

G. Edlin and E. Golanty (1992), *Health and Wellness,* Boston: Jones and Bartlett Publishers. Reprinted by permission.

with life changes constructively by doing the following.

1. Consider what the change means to you personally.

2. Consider the change's meaning in your life and focus on your feelings about it.

3. Examine and explore alternatives for adjusting to the change.

4. Think it through before acting — a measured response is usually better than an impulsive one.

5. Pace yourself. Frenetic activity leads to ineffectiveness, and it is a drain on one's energy reserve.

6. Engage in relaxation activities such as exercise, voluntary relaxation techniques, or other enjoyable activities such as a movie, concert, a picnic, an outing.

7. Follow a regular daily routine as closely as possible.

8. Talk to family and friends who can be a source of support as well as objective observers who may be able to offer alternative solutions.

There are two categories of stress: acute and chronic. Acute stress is situational and of short duration. It is the type of stress associated with taking exams or interviewing for a job or changing jobs, or moving to a new apartment. Physiological responses to such events occur immediately before as well as during the event. These include an increase in the secretion of epinephrine which accelerates resting heart rate and blood pressure, increases the blood supply to the muscles and decreases it to the digestive system and kidneys, dilates the pupils of the eyes to take in more information, increases blood sugar level, and slightly depresses the immune system. The stressor loses its effect when the event is over, allowing these physiological responses to return to normal. However, if stress is chronic, or long-lasting, it prolongs the responses and these changes represent a significant strain on the body. Examples of chronic stress include the necessity of having to make quotas and deadlines, or working in a job where the employee feels a loss of control, or that one's input is not valued. If people cannot physically or psychologically adapt or separate themselves from the stressor, the ability to resist weakens. Months or years of interacting with a stressor depletes the body's adaptive ability. At this point, professional counseling and medication may be needed to get through the long rehabilitation process required to return the individual to normal.

Several techniques and methods are available for controlling stress. However, we will concentrate specifically on the contribution of exercise. Many studies have indicated that physically fit people subjected to laboratory induced psychosocial stress exhibit a reduced response to those stressors when compared to unfit people. Additionally, they recover from stress more rapidly and are less vulnerable to stress-related diseases. Vulnerability to disease is decreased probably due to a more robust immune system that can ward off infectious diseases and is more efficient in recognizing and destroying mutant cells. Some authorities attribute our enhanced disease fighting capability, in part, to the pyrogenic effect of exercise. The increased body temperature during and immediately after exercise simulates, on a temporary basis, the fever produced naturally by the body in response to viral and bacterial infections. This represents one of the body's defense mechanisms for counteracting disease.

Another explanation for the feeling of well-being experienced by physically active people is that exercise increases the production of endogenous opiates (primarily the beta endorphins) that elevate mood, give relief from pain, and provide feelings of relaxation. Finally, exercise reduces blood levels of the catecholamines (epinephrine and norepinephrine) that raise blood pressure by increasing peripheral vascular resistance.

Exercise is beneficial for both body and mind because it produces positive physiological and personality changes. People who lose fat and gain muscle become more satisfied with their physical appearance and as such, they experience a lift in self-esteem.

Exercise is a stressor but one that is concrete, easily identifiable, and during participation it replaces ambiguous or nonspecific psychosocial stress. It is also an outlet for the release of pent up energy.

Depression

Clinical depression is prolonged sadness that persists beyond a reasonable length of time. The symptoms include social withdrawal, feelings of helplessness, and loss of control of one's life. Exercise is accepted as one component in a spectrum of treatments for depression.[18] Studies have shown that aerobic exercises, primarily walking and jogging, have improved the mental health status of depressed patients. Many of these patients improved dramatically enough to be taken off medication while the improvement of others led to a reduction in medications. The patients who exercised the most improved the most.

Summary

- Cancer is the second leading cause of death in the U.S.
- Cancer is characterized by abnormal and uncontrollable cellular growth.
- Oncogenes are cancerous genes.
- Exercise helps to prevent cancer by reducing body fat, stimulating the immune system, and by increasing the transit of food through the digestive system.
- Osteoporosis is a silent disease characterized by the gradual loss of bone mass.
- Women are affected by osteoporosis more often and at an earlier age than men.
- The risk factors for osteoporosis include age, gender, heredity, lack of physical activity, cigarette smoking, and insufficient calcium intake.
- Osteoporosis is treatable but not curable.
- Weight bearing aerobic exercises and weight training exercise are best for developing and maintaining the skeletal system.
- Osteoarthritis is the result of wear of the cartilage between joints.
- The major cause of osteoarthritis is obesity.
- Exercise is important because it lubricates and nourishes the joints.
- Nonweight-bearing exercises, such as water sports and activities, can be used if land-based weight-bearing exercises cause pain.
- There are 5000 asthma-related deaths annually in the U.S.
- The American Academy of Allergy and Immunology encourages asthmatics to exercise regularly.
- Exercised-induced asthma occurs from the loss of respiratory heat and water due to high breathing rates.
- Swimming and other water activities are the least asthmogenic of the many forms of exercise.

▶ Stress is the nonspecific response of the human organism to any demand, positive or negative, that it encounters.

▶ The individual's response or reaction to a stressor rather than the stressor itself, will determine its impact.

▶ There are two kinds of stress: acute and chronic.

▶ Acute stress is situational and of short duration while chronic stress is long term and potentially harmful.

▶ Physically fit people have a reduced response to stress, recover more rapidly, and are less vulnerable to stress-related diseases.

▶ Physically fit people develop a more robust immune system, they may have higher levels of endorphins, and they have lower circulating catecholamine levels.

▶ Clinical depression, (prolonged sadness that persists beyond a reasonable length of time) responds to exercise that is performed on a regular basis.

▶ # REFERENCES

1. *Cancer Facts and Figures - 1994*, Atlanta, GA: American Cancer Society, 1994.

2. Simon, H. B. "Can You Run Away From Cancer?," *Harvard Health Letter*, 17: (March, 1992), p. 5.

3. "Does Exercise Protect Against Cancer?" *University of California at Berkeley Wellness Letter*, 9: (November, 1992), p. 6.

4. Frisch, R. E., "Lower Prevalence of Breast Cancer and Cancers of the Reproductive System Among Former College Athletes Compared to Non-Athletes," *British Journal of Cancer*, 52: (1985), p. 885.

5. "Boosting Your Immune System" *University of California at Berkeley Wellness Letter*, 10: (October, 1993), p. 4.

6. "A Lifelong Program to Build Strong Bones." *University of California at Berkeley Wellness Letter*, 9: (July, 1993), p. 4.

7. Rankin, J. W. and Volpe, S. L. "Diet, Exercise, and Osteoporosis," *ASCM Certified News*, 3: (December, 1993), p. 1.

8. "A Lifelong Program to Build Strong Bones."

9. Rankin, J. W., et al., "Diet, Exercise, and Osteoporosis."

10. Schardt, D. "These Feet Were Made For Walking" *Nutrition Action Health Letter*, 20: (December, 1993), p. 1.

11. Conroy, B. P. et al, "Adaptive Responses of Bone to Physical Activity," *Medicine, Exercise, Nutrition, and Health*, 1: (1992), p. 64.

12. "Exercise and Arthritis: The Importance of a Regular Program." *University of California at Berkeley Wellness Letter*, 10: (April, 1994), p. 6.

13. Felson, D. T. "Obesity and Knee Osteoarthritis. The Framingham Study," *Annals of Internal Medicine* 109: (1988), p. 18.

14 National Asthma Education Program, Expert Panel Report. *Guidelines for the Diagnosis and Management of Asthma*, Bethesda, MD: Office of Prevention, Education, and Control, National Heart, Lung, and Blood Institute, National Institutes of Health, (Publication No. 91-3042), August, 1991.

15. Sabath, R. J. "Exercise - Induced Asthma in Children and Adolescents," *ACSM Certified News* 4: (April, 1994), p. 5.

16. Mahler, D. "Exercise - Induced Asthma," *Medicine and Science in Sports and Exercise*, 25: (May, 1993), p. 554.

17. Afrasiabi, R. and Spector, S. L. "Exercise-Induced Asthma," *The Physician and Sportsmedicine* 19: (May, 1991), p. 49.

18. Raglin, J. "Exercise and Mental Health: Beneficial and Detrimental Effects," *Sports Medicine*, 9: (1990), p. 323.

Nutrition for Active People

This chapter covers two important factors, (1) the basics of a nutritious diet, and (2) the effects of diet and exercise on weight control. Carbohydrates, fats, protein, vitamins, minerals, and water are the basic nutrients that allow the body to perform its many functions. This includes fuel for muscle contraction, the maintenance and repair of the body's tissues, the regulation of chemical reactions at the cellular level, the transmission of neural impulses, and the growth and reproduction of cells.

This chapter also covers the role of diet and exercise in weight control. The contributions and limitations of each are also discussed. Selected techniques for measuring overweight and overfat are also presented.

BASIC NUTRITION

Metabolism is the sum total of chemical reactions whereby the energy liberated from food is made available to the body. Two processes are involved: (1) anabolism — substances are built into new tissues or stored in some form for later use, and (2) catabolism — the breakdown of complex materials to simpler ones for the release of energy for muscular contraction.

Catabolism occurs when food is combined with oxygen. This process, referred to as oxidation, transforms food materials into heat or mechanical energy. The energy value of food is expressed in calories. In this text, we will deal with the large calorie (Kcal) which is the amount of heat needed to increase the temperature of one kilogram of water (slightly more than one quart) by one degree centigrade. This is sometimes referred to as the nutritionist's calorie in that it is the unit that is commonly used to assign the caloric value to food.

THE FOOD GUIDE PYRAMID

In 1992, the U.S. Department of Agriculture released the Food Guide Pyramid. This replaces the basic four food groups and is a significant step forward in directing this nation's attention toward healthier eating, (See Figure 7.1) The most desirable foods from a health perspective are the breads, cereals, pastas, fruits, and vegetables that are located at the base of the pyramid, while the least desirable (fats, oils, and sweets) are located at the apex. Each level is accompanied by suggestions for the number of daily servings that should be consumed.

The Food Guide Pyramid is a very useful guide, but it contains some deficiencies. For example, (1) there is no mention of how large a serving should be, (2) dry beans should not be in the third level with meat because of the significant difference in fat content between the two, (3) there is no mention of skim milk dairy products, and (4) it does not differentiate between saturated and unsaturated fat. Barring these criticisms, its development has been a worthwhile effort.

Food Guide Pyramid
A Guide to Daily Food Choices

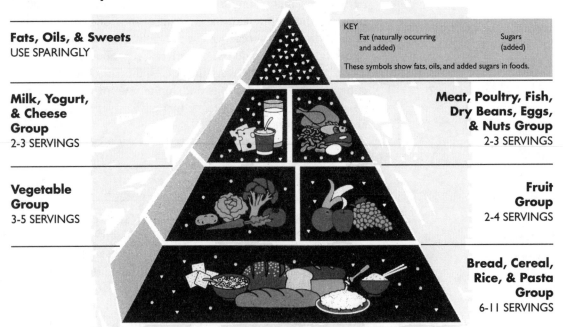

Figure 7.1   The Food Guide Pyramid: A Guide to Daily Food Choices.

The New Food Labels

By May, 1994 all processed foods should display the new labels mandated by the federal government. The new labels are a substantial improvement over the old ones in that they will facilitate the comparison of foods based on nutritional quantity and quality. The upper half of the new label describes the nutritional information related specifically to the food in the package, while the lower half will be constant for all food products

The upper half of the label provides the percent daily value for six important nutrients. The food label in Figure 7.2 indicates that the total fat in this food represents five percent of the daily allowance but the sodium content of this item represents 13% of the daily allowance. The information on the upper half of the label can assist consumers in planning their daily menu without exceeding the nutritional recommendations for a given day. It also allows them to select the best foods by comparing several for caloric content as well as basic nutrients.

The lower half provides the upper limit for selected nutrients for diets consisting of either 2000 Kcals or 2500 Kcals. Adjustments to these values should be made if your calorie intake is higher or lower.

The Calorie Containing Nutrients

Carbohydrates

Carbohydrates (CHO) are organic compounds composed of one or more sugars (saccharides) which are derived from plants. Carbohydrates consist of monosaccharides (simple sugar), disaccharides (combination of two simple sugars), and polysaccharides (the joining of three or more simple sugars to form starch and glycogen).

Table sugar, corn syrup, molasses, and honey are examples of simple sugars. Americans,

---

Nutrition facts
Serving size 1/2 cup (114 g)
Servings per container 4

Amount per serving

Calories 90   Calories from fat 30

	Percent Daily Value *
Total fat 3 g	5%
Saturated fat 0 g	0%
Cholesterol 0 mg	0%
Sodium 30 mg	13%
Total carbohydrate 13 g	4%
Dietary fiber 3 g	12%
Sugars 3 g	
Protein 3 g	

Vitamin A	80%	Vitamin C	60%
Calcium	4%	Iron	4%

*Percent Daily Values are based on a 2,000 calorie diet. Your daily values may be higher or lower depending on your calorie needs:

		Calories	2,000	2,500
Total fat	Less than		65 g	80 g
Saturated fat	Less than		20 g	25 g
Cholesterol	Less than		300 mg	300 mg
Sodium	Less than		2,400 mg	2,400 mg
Total carbohydrate			300 g	375 g
Fiber			25 g	30 g

Calories per gram:
Fat   9   Carbohydrates   4   Protein   4

Figure 7.2   The new food label.

---

active and inactive, consume too much of these substances. It is estimated that Americans spend more than $9 billion per year on sweeteners — 85% of this total is for sugar, the remaining 15% is for artificial sweeteners.[1] The annual per capita consumption of sugar in the U.S. is 136 lbs. plus another 20 lbs. of artificial sweetener on top of that. Most of this is in the form of hidden sugar; that is, it is included in processed foods. Canned soups and vegetables, canned meats, cereal, dairy products, soft drinks and many other items are laden with sugar. Simple sugars are called "empty calories" because they are rich in calories but provide little or no nutrition.

Many authorities feel that the excessive consumption of simple sugars leads to obesity, Type II diabetes, elevated cholesterol, heart disease, and dental caries. But, the evidence does not support most of these assumptions.[2] According to the American Dietetic Association, sugar has been erroneously indicted as the cause of a number of health problems.[3] Sugar is not an independent risk factor for any disease except in the case of a few rare heredity disorders. It is however, a major cause of tooth decay. Sugar should constitute less than 10% of the total calories. (See Figure 7.3)

The bulk of carbohydrates consumed should come from the complex variety. These include starch and several forms of fiber. The complex carbohydrates are nutrient dense for the number of calories they contain. This category of food is precisely what weight and health conscious people need. Today's dictum for health

and weight control is "lower the fat content of the diet." Increasing the complex carbohydrate intake is a painless way to do this. Eating starchy foods — grains, legumes, tubers, and pastas — is not only healthy, but tasty. All starches come from plant foods, most of which contain only trace amounts of fat. There are some exceptions such as olives, avocados, nuts, seeds, coconuts, etc. that contain substantial amounts of fat. These should be consumed in moderation.

A diet high in fresh plant foods will also be high in fiber. But if plant products are processed or refined, the quantity of fiber will be diminished significantly, if not totally removed. There are two types of dietary fiber: soluble which dissolves in hot water, and insoluble which does not dissolve. Both are beneficial to health but in different ways. Both are indigestible polysaccharides found in the stems, leaves, and seeds of plants.

Soluble fiber adds bulk to the contents of the stomach. This slows stomach emptying and prolongs the sense of feeling full. This is good for weight watchers. Soluble fiber also lowers blood cholesterol levels. Reducing body weight

Food Category	Current Consumption (% of total Kcals)	Recommended Consumption (% of total Kcals)
Carbohydrates (CHO)	48% a. 1/2 Sugar b. 1/2 Complex CHO	58% a. < 10% Sugar * b. 48% Complex CHO
Fat	37–38% a. 17–18% Saturated b. 20% Unsaturated	a. < 10% Saturated b. 10% Monounsaturated c. 10% Polyunsaturated
Protein	15%	12%

* < means less than

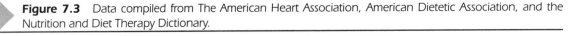 **Figure 7.3** Data compiled from The American Heart Association, American Dietetic Association, and the Nutrition and Diet Therapy Dictionary.

and cholesterol lowers the risk of cardiovascular disease.

Insoluble fiber adds bulk to the contents of the intestines thus accelerating the passage of food remnants through the digestive tract. This has several healthy effects: (1) it decreases the time for tissue exposure to toxins and carcinogenic substances thereby providing some protection against colon cancer, (2) it prevents or alleviates constipation, and (3) it stimulates muscle tone in the intestinal walls that increases resistance to diverticulosis (a condition of saclike swellings in the wall of the intestines). Most plants contain some of both types of fiber. Good sources of fiber are found in Table 7.1.

When oxidized, carbohydrates yield approximately four calories per gram. Because they are oxygen rich, they constitute our most efficient source of fuel. They are the major energy supplier in high intensity work of short duration and in exercise of a vigorous nature for up to sixty to ninety minutes.

Foods high in carbohydrates promote the storage of glycogen (the stored form of sugar) in the liver and muscles. Increasing the storage of glycogen enhances aerobic performance of long duration such as marathon running and long distance cycling. People who do not run such long distances should consume a diet rich in complex carbohydrates primarily because it is a healthy way to eat. Active adults should consume about 48% of their calories in the form of complex carbohydrates and no more that ten percent in the form of simple sugar. People who train for and compete in prolonged endurance events should consume sixty-five to seventy percent of their calories from the carbohydrate group.

Fats

Fats are energy dense organic compounds that yield approximately 9 calories per gram.

Table 7.1 Selected Sources of Fiber

	DIETARY FIBER (gm)
1. Cereals	
100% Bran (½ cup)	8.4
All Bran (½ cup)	8.5
Bran Buds (⅓ cup)	7.9
Bran Chex (⅔ cup)	4.6
Corn Bran (⅔ cup)	5.4
Cracklin' Oat Bran (⅓ cup)	4.3
Bran Flakes (¾ cup)	4.0
Oatmeal, cooked (1 cup)	2.2
2. Grains (1 ounce)	
Brown rice, cooked (½ cup)	2.4
Millet, cooked (½ cup)	1.8
Whole wheat bread (1 slice)	1.0
Spaghetti, cooked (½ cup)	0.8
White bread (1 slice)	0.6
White rice, cooked (½ cup)	0.1
3. Legumes (½ cup)	
Kidney beans	5.8
Pinto beans	5.3
Split peas	5.1
White beans	5.0
Lima beans	4.9
4. Vegetables (½ cup)	
Sweet potato (1 large)	4.2
Peas	4.1
Brussels sprouts	3.9
Corn	3.9
Potato, baked (1 medium)	3.8
Carrots (1 raw; ½ cup cooked)	2.3
Collards	2.2
Asparagus	2.1
Green beans	2.1
Broccoli	2.0
Spinach	2.0
Turnips	1.7
Mushrooms (raw)	0.9
Summer squash	0.7
Lettuce (raw)	0.3
5. Fruits	
Blackberries (½ cup)	4.5
Prunes, dried (3)	3.7
Apples with skin (1)	2.6
Banana (1 medium)	2.0
Strawberries (¾ cup)	2.0
Grapefruit (½ med)	1.7
Peach (1 med)	1.6
Cantaloupe (¼ small)	1.4
Raisins (2 tablespoons)	1.3
Orange (1 small)	1.2
Grapes (12)	0.5

Adapted from J. Anderson, *Plant Fiber in Foods*, Lexington, KY: HFC Diabetes Research Foundation, Inc., 1986; *Nutrition Action Health-letter* (April 1986); and E. Lanza and R. R. Butram, "A Critical Review of Food Fiber Analysis and Data," *Journal of the American Dietetic Association* 86 (1986): 732.

They have a relatively low oxygen content when compared to carbohydrates and consequently are not as efficient as sources of fuel. It takes more than twice the amount of oxygen to liberate energy from fat than from carbohydrates. But we store at least fifty times more energy in the form of fat than as carbohydrates. A pound of fat as it is stored in the body contains 3500 Kcals.

The triglycerides are the most abundant of the fats (lipids). The triglycerides make-up at least 95% of the fat that is consumed as well as that which is stored. Triglycerides are composed of three fatty acids attached to a molecule of glycerol. Fatty acids are classified as saturated or unsaturated, based upon their chemical structure. A fatty acid is a long chain of carbon atoms (C) bonded to hydrogen atoms (H), with an acid group at the end of the molecule. Fatty acids are saturated when all of the bonds between the carbon atoms are single bonds (see Figure 7.4a). Monounsaturated fatty acids have one double bond between carbon atoms (see Figure 7.4b). Polyunsaturated fatty acids have two or more double bonds between the carbon atoms (see Figure 7.4c).

The major source of saturated fats are animal flesh, dairy products, and tropical oils (coconut, palm kernel oil). Saturated fats have a high melting point and solidify at room temperature. Bacon or sausage grease that stands at room temperature will solidify, signifying that it is saturated. Monounsaturated and polyunsaturated fats remain liquid at room temperature. Some food sources that are high in monounsaturated fats are avocados, canola oil, cashew nuts, olives, olive oil, peanuts, peanut oil, and peanut butter. Polyunsaturated fats are found in almonds, corn oil, cottonseed oil, filbert nuts, fish, pecan, safflower oil, sunflower oil, soybean oil, and walnuts. Some sources of plant-derived cooking oils appear in Table 7.2.

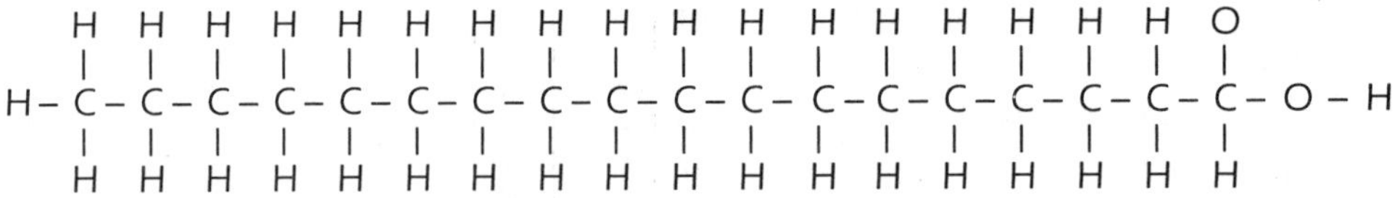

(a) Saturated fatty acid — no double bonds: all carbons are occupied.

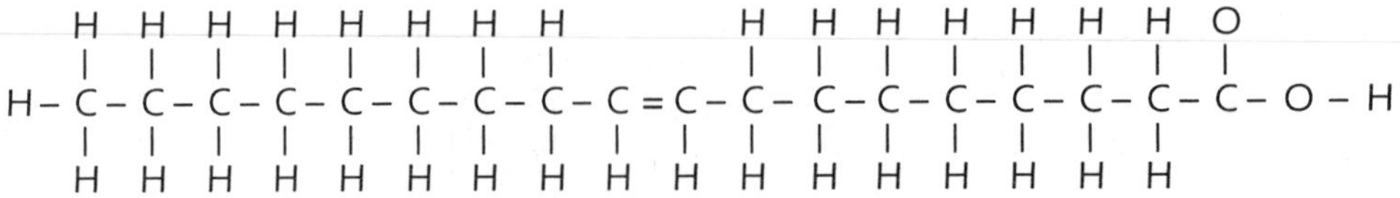

(b) Monounsaturated fatty acid — one double bond; two hydrogens missing at that site.

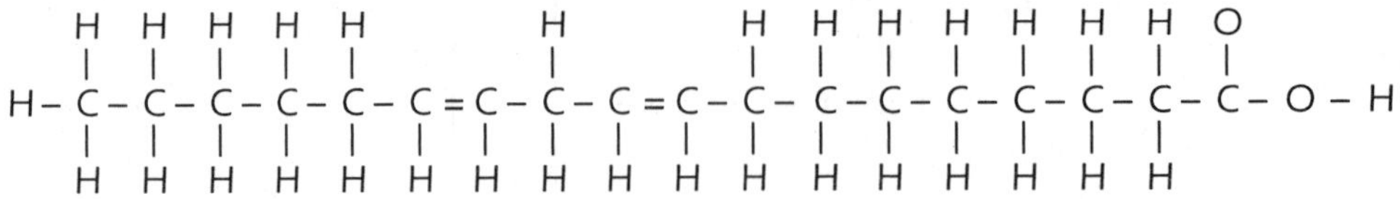

(c) Polyunsaturated fatty acid — two double bonds; four hydrogen missing at the site.

Figure 7.4 Different types of fatty acids.

▶ **Table 7.2** Some Sources of Plant-Derived Cooking Oils

Type of Oil	Monounsaturated (grams)	Polyunsaturated (grams)	Saturated (grams)
Best Sources			
Almond	10	2	1
Canola	8	4	1
Olive	10	1	2
Good Sources			
Corn	3	8	2
Cottonseed	2	7	4
Safflower	2	10	1
Sesame	5	6	2
Soybean	3	8	2
Sunflower	3	9	1

1 gram = 1/28 ounce.

Fatty acids derived from fish, especially cold water fish, are different from those found in vegetables and vegetable oils. The fatty acids in fish are Omega-3s while those found in vegetables are primarily Omega-6s. Omega-3 fatty acids protect the heart and its blood vessels by decreasing the likelihood that the blood platelets will stick to each other. Decreasing that possibility reduces plaque build-up, clot formation, and spasms occurring in the arteries.[4]

Trans fatty acids

Unsaturated fats should be refrigerated to keep them from becoming rancid. They are vulnerable to spoilage when left to stand at room temperature because oxygen attacks those points in the chain that are unoccupied by hydrogen. To counteract spoilage, the food industry adds hydrogen to some of the free bonds through the process of hydrogenation. The fat then loses its polyunsaturated characteristics as well its health benefits. Hydrogenation converts many double bonds to single bonds. The end product is the conversion of unsaturated fatty acids to trans fatty acids. Margarine is the major source of trans fatty acids in the American diet.

Vegetable oils are liquid and must be made more saturated if they are to be solidified into margarine. The harder the product (stick margarine) — versus softer margarines (tub and squeeze bottle) — the greater the effect of hydrogenation. The question to be answered is, Does the conversion of unsaturated fatty acids to trans fatty acids result in an unhealthy product? Recent evidence indicates that trans fatty acids have an effect similar to the saturated fats, that is, they raise the blood level of harmful LDL cholesterol.[5] Unfortunately, the new food labels do not record the grams of trans fatty acids that are found in processed foods.

Eating a fat-free diet is virtually impossible and definitely unhealthy. The human body requires some fat. There are two important fatty acids that are essential — they must be obtained through the diet because they cannot be manufactured from other substances in the body. Both are polyunsaturated fatty acids that are widely distributed in plant and fish oils. Linoleic acid is an Omega-6 fatty acid found in plants, while the second, linoleic fatty acid is an Omega-3 found primarily in fish.

Proteins

Protein is an essential nutrient that yields approximately 4 calories per gram. Its energy is liberated for building and repairing body tissues; forming enzymes, hormones, antibodies, and hemoglobin; transporting fats and other nutrients through the blood; maintaining acid-base balance in tissue fluids; and supplying energy for muscular work when there is a shortage of carbohydrates and fat.

Proteins are complex chemical structures containing carbon, oxygen, hydrogen, and nitrogen. These elements are combined into chains of different structures called amino acids. There is general agreement that the proteins of all living tissue consist of 20 different amino acids. Two other rare amino acids have been identified but are found in very few proteins. Nine of the amino acids are essential because they cannot be manufactured in the body and can only be obtained through the diet. Complete proteins — those containing all the essential amino acids — are found in meat, fish, poultry, and dairy products. The proteins found in vegetables and cereal grains generally do not contain all of the essential amino acids, but complementary foods from these two groups may be selected so that one supplies those amino acids missing in the other. See Table 7.3 for combinations of food that together provide complete proteins.

Legumes, such as kidney and lima beans, black-eyed peas, garden peas, lentils, and soybeans, are excellent sources of proteins. Although their protein is not quite the caliber of meat protein, they are rich in other healthy nutrients such as B vitamins, and they are low in fat.

Daily protein requirements vary according to one's position in the life cycle. Infants require about 2.2 grams of protein per kilogram of body weight to support growth. Adolescents require 1.0 gram per kilogram, and adults need 0.8 gram per kilogram.

The typical American diet contains more than adequate amounts of protein. There seems to be no advantage in consuming more than 12 percent of the total calories in the form of protein. One of the major problems associated with excessive protein intake is that it is usually accomplished by increasing the consumption of animal products, which are also high in saturated fat. This increased consumption may displace fiber in the diet and the

TABLE 7.3   Vegetable Combinations That Provide Complete Proteins

CATEGORIES OF FOODS	EXAMPLES
Beans/wheat	Baked beans and brown bread
Beans/rice	Refried beans and rice
Dry peas/rye	Split pea soup and rye bread
Peanut butter/wheat	Peanut butter sandwich on whole wheat or whole grain bread
Cornmeal/beans	Cornbread and kidney beans
Legumes/rice	Black-eyed peas and rice
Beans/corn	Pinto beans and cornbread
Legumes/corn	Black-eyed peas and cornbread

Adapted from A. C. Grandjeans. *The Vegetarian Athlete* 15 (1987): 191.

two together can lead to a host of immediate and long-term problems.

The average daily consumption of protein by adults in the U.S. is about 15% of the total calories. This amount is well above the requirement. For example, a 154 lb. person requires 56 grams of protein each day, but, if this person is consuming 2500 Kcals/day with a typical protein intake of 15%, this person would actually be consuming 94 grams of protein. These figures come from the following:

1. Protein requirement is calculated as follows:

   a. convert body weight in lbs. to kilograms (kg)

   $$\frac{154}{2.2} = 70\ kg$$

   b. 70 kg × .8 grams = 56 grams/day

2. Actual consumption is calculated as follows:

   a.   2500   Kcals/day
         × .15   percentage of protein in the diet
          375   Kcals of protein

   b. One gram of protein yields 4 Kcals therefore

   $$\frac{375\ g\ of\ protein}{4\ grams} = 94\ grams\ of\ protein$$

   c. The difference between protein consumed and protein required is:

        94 consumed
      −54 required
        38 extra grams of protein

Many people — competitors and noncompetitors alike — who are striving to develop strength and power have been taking amino acid supplements to build larger and more powerful muscles. Selected amino acids do not build larger muscles; only exercise can do that. However, these and other unfounded notions proliferate among uninformed participants who are constantly attempting to enhance performance with substances that might give them an edge beyond that achieved with training. Current evidence indicates that long distance endurance-type athletes have the greatest need for protein. They need 1.5 to 1.6 grams of protein for every kilogram of body weight.[6] Even if this proves to be correct, protein supplements are not necessary, since most athletes consume more than this amount from their food intake. Suppose a 145 lb marathon runner consumes 4,800 Kcals/day. His protein intake represents 15 percent of his total calories. How many grams of protein does he consume, and how many does he actually need if his requirement is 1½ times the normal amount for adults?

1. Convert body weight in pounds to kilograms (kg)

   $$\frac{145\ lbs.}{2.2} = 66\ kg$$

2.   4,800 Kcals consumed
     × .15 percentage of protein in diet
        720 Kcals/protein

3. 1 gram of protein yields 4 Kcals; therefore,

   $$\frac{720}{4} = 180\ grams\ protein\ intake$$

4. Protein required is 1.6 grams per kg of body weight

       66 Kg
    × 1.6
    105.6 grams

5. Difference between protein consumed and protein required:

      180 consumed
    −106 needed
       74 grams of extra protein

In light of the preceding example, protein supplementation or amino acid supplements are unnecessary and a waste of money.

The Non-Calorie-Containing Nutrients

Vitamins

Vitamins are noncaloric organic compounds found in small quantities in most foods. All vitamins are either fat soluble or water soluble. The fat-soluble vitamins (A,D,E, and K) are stored in the liver and fatty tissues until they are needed. The water-soluble vitamins (C and the B complex group) are not stored for any appreciable length of time and must be replenished daily.

Vitamins function as coenzymes that promote the many chemical reactions that occur in the body around the clock. Since vitamin deficiencies result in a variety of diseases, and adequate daily intake is necessary, the recommended daily allowances (RDA) have been established for most vitamins. Although these amounts are needed to prevent the occurrence of diseases that are the result of vitamin deficiencies, they do not represent optimal values. Today, the interest in vitamins by the scientific community goes beyond that. For instance, a substantial research effort is currently in progress as investigators attempt to clarify the role of selected antioxidant vitamins (C, E, and beta carotene) in the prevention of cardiovascular disease and cancer. The early evidence is promising and these vitamins appear to be safe even when taken in larger amounts than recommended.

However, unusually large doses (megadosing) of any vitamin might be potentially hazardous. Those who supplement heavily may experience vitamin toxicity, particularly from overindulgence in the fat-soluble group. When vitamins are taken in very large amounts, they cease to function as vitamins and begin to act like drugs. Also, large doses interfere or disrupt the action of other nutrients. See Tables 7.4 and 7.5 for problems associated with vitamin megadoses.

Table 7.4 Toxic Symptoms — Fat Soluble Vitamins

Vitamin (U.S. RDA)	Sources	Toxic Symptoms
Vitamin A * (1000 mg)	Fortified milk and margarine, cream, cheese, butter, eggs, liver, spinach and other dark leafy greens, broccoli, apricots, peaches, cantaloupe, squash, carrots, sweet potatoes, and pumpkin.	Red blood cell breakage, nosebleeds, abdominal cramps, nausea, diarrhea, weight loss, blurred vision, irritability, loss of appetite, bone pain, dry skin, rashes, hair loss, cessation of menstruation, growth retardation.
Vitamin D ** (400 IU)	Self-synthesis with sunlight, fortified milk, fortified margarine, eggs, liver, fish.	Raised blood calcium, constipation, weight loss, irritability, weakness, nausea, kidney stones, mental and physical retardation.
Vitamin E (30 IU)	Vegetable oils, green leafy vegetables, wheat germ, whole-grain products, butter, liver, egg yolk, milk fat, nuts, seeds.	Interference with anticlotting medication, general discomfort.
Vitamin K (no U.S. RDA)	Bacterial synthesis in digestive tract, liver, green leafy and cruciferous vegetables, milk.	Interference with anticlotting medication; may cause jaundice.

*   mg = micrograms
** IU = international units

> **Table 7.5** Toxic Symptoms — Water Soluble Vitamins

Vitamin (U.S. RDA)	Sources	Toxic Symptoms
Thiamin B$_1$ * (1.5 mg)	Meat, pork, liver, fish, poultry, whole-grain and enriched breads, cereals, pasta, nuts, legumes, wheat germ, oats	Rapid pulse, weakness, headaches, insomnia, irritability
Riboflavin B$_2$ (1.7 mg)	Milk, dark green vegetables, yogurt, cottage cheese, liver, meat, whole-grain or enriched breads and cereals	None reported, but an excess of any of the B vitamins could cause a deficiency of the others
Niacin B$_3$ (20 mg)	Meat, eggs, poultry, fish, milk, whole-grain and enriched breads and cereals, nuts, legumes, peanuts, nutritional yeast, all protein foods	Flushing, nausea, headaches, cramps, ulcer irritation, heartburn, abnormal liver function, low blood pressure
Vitamin B$_6$ (2.0 mg)	Meat, poultry, fish, shellfish, legumes, whole-grain products, green leafy vegetables, bananas	Depression, fatigue, irritability, headaches, numbness, damage to nerves, difficulty walking
Folcain (Folic acid) (400 micrograms)	Green leafy vegetables, organ meats, legumes, seeds	Diarrhea, insomnia, irritability; may mask a vitamin B$_{12}$ deficiency
Vitamin B$_{12}$ **(cobalamin) (3 g)	Animal products: meats, fish, poultry, shellfish, milk, cheese, eggs, nutritional yeast	None reported
Pantothenic acid (10 mg)	Widespread in foods	Occasional diarrhea
Biotin (300 g)	Widespread in foods	None reported
Vitamin C (Ascorbic acid) (60 mg)	Citrus fruits, cruciferous vegetables, tomatoes, potatoes, dark green vegetables, peppers, lettuce, cantaloupe, strawberries, mangos, papayas	Nausea, abdominal cramps, diarrhea, breakdown of red blood cells in persons with certain genetic disorders: deficiency symptoms may appear at first on withdrawal of high doses

*   mg = micrograms
** g = grams

Are synthetic vitamin supplements inferior to natural vitamin supplements? Promoters of vitamin products that come from natural sources adamantly proclaim that this is correct but in reality the synthetic and natural supplements are chemically equivalent and the body cannot tell them apart. The manufacturers and vendors, rather than the consumers, are the beneficiaries of the sale of natural vitamins because they are substantially more expensive and their profit margin is greater. So don't be fooled by this old gambit. And remember, the best sources of vitamins come from the foods that we eat.

Active people get more vitamins in their diet than sedentary people because they consume more calories. If you are concerned about not getting enough vitamins in your diet but are unwilling to make appropriate dietary changes, a one-a-day brand should do. More than this amount is unnecessary and costly.

Minerals

Minerals are inorganic substances that exist freely in nature. They are found in the earth's soil and water, and they pervade some of the earth's vegetation. Minerals maintain or regulate such physiological processes as muscle contraction, normal heart rhythm, body water supplies, acid-base balance of the blood, and nerve impulse conduction. Calcium, phosphorous, potassium, sulphur, sodium, chloride, and magnesium are the major minerals. They are classified as major because they occur in the body in quantities greater than five grams. The trace minerals, or micronutrients, number a dozen or more. The distinction between the major and trace minerals is one of quantity rather than importance. Deficiencies of either can have serious consequences.

Sodium, potassium, and chloride are the primary minerals lost through perspiration. Sodium, the positive ion in sodium chloride (table salt), is one of the body's major electrolytes (ions that conduct electricity). Americans consume three to four grams of sodium daily, but only 1.8 to 2.4 grams are recommended.[7] Approximately 70 percent of the salt consumed in the United States is located in processed foods such as canned and instant soups, smoked meats and fish, cheeses, and deep-fried snacks. Salt is a cheap preservative and flavor enhancer. Read the labels on all canned and packaged foods to get an idea of the amount of salt that the product contains. The other 30% of our salt intake results from using the salt shaker and from naturally occurring salt in the foods we eat.

Sodium is found in the fluid outside of the cells, while potassium is found within cellular fluid. The temporary exchange of sodium and potassium across the cell's membrane permits the transmission of neural impulses and the contraction of muscles. Low potassium levels interfere with muscle cell nutrition and lead to muscle weakness and fatigue. Potassium is essential for the maintenance of the heartbeat. Starvation and very low calorie diets for prolonged periods can produce sudden death from heart failure as potassium storage drops to critically low levels. Vomiting, diarrhea, and diuretics (substances to rid the body of excess water) reduce potassium levels. Chronic physical activity that produces heavy sweating probably will not diminish potassium stores unless the diet is woefully lacking in this mineral. It is hard to reduce potassium stores because potassium is contained in most foods and is easily replaced. It is particularly abundant in citrus fruits and juices, bananas, dates, nuts, fresh vegetables, meat, and fish.

As with vitamins, mineral intake can be abused. Excess amounts of both major and trace minerals produce a variety of symptoms (see Tables 7.6 and 7.7).

Water

People can survive for a month or more without food, but a few days without water will result in death. Since all body processes and chemical reactions take place in a liquid medium, it is imperative to be fully hydrated and to make a special effort to replace water when it is lost. Under normal conditions, adults drink 1.2 to 1.4 liters of fluid each day. More is needed when the weather is hot and humid or when one is physically active regardless of weather conditions.

Approximately 40% to 60% of the body's weight consists of water. A sizable amount is stored in the muscles, and some is stored in fat. By virtue of his larger muscle mass, the average male stores more water than the average female. Sixty-two percent of the total amount is found in the intracellular compartment (water within the cells), while the remaining 38 percent is extracellular (water in the blood, lymph system, spinal cord fluid, saliva, etc.)

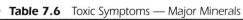

Table 7.6   Toxic Symptoms — Major Minerals

Minerals (U.S. RDA)	Selected Sources	Toxic Symptoms
Calcium, Phosphorus (1000 mg)	Calcium: milk and milk products, small fish (with bones), tofu, greens, legumes, Phosphorus: all animal tissues	Excess calcium is excreted except in hormonal imbalance states. Excess phosphorus can cause relative deficiency of calcium
Magnesium (400 mg)	Nuts, legumes, whole grains, dark green vegetables, seafoods, chocolate, cocoa	Not known
Sodium (no U.S. RDA)	Salt, soy sauce, moderate quantities in whole (unprocessed), foods, large amounts in processed foods	Hypertension
Chloride (no U.S. RDA)	Salt, soy sauce, moderate quantities in whole (unprocessed), foods, large amounts in processed foods	Normally harmless (the gas chlorine is a poison but evaporates from water), disturbed acid-base balance, vomiting
Potassium (no U.S. RDA)	All whole foods: meats, milk, fruits, vegetables, grains, legumes	Causes muscular weakness, triggers vomiting; if given into a vein, can stop the heart
Sulfur (no U.S. RDA)	All protein-containing foods	Would occur only if sulfur amino acids were eaten in excess; this (in animals) depresses growth

Table 7.7   Toxic Symptoms — Trace Minerals

Minerals (U.S. RDA)	Sources	Toxic Symptoms
Iodine (150 g)	Iodized salt, seafood	Very high intakes depress thyroid activity
Iron (18 mg)	Red meats, fish, poultry, shellfish, eggs, legumes, dried fruits	Iron overload: infections, liver injury
Zinc (15 mg)	Protein-containing foods: meats, fish, poultry, grains, vegetables	Fever, nausea, vomiting, diarrhea
Copper (2 mg)	Meats, drinking water	Unknown except as part of a rare hereditary disease (Wilson's disease)
Fluoride (no U.S. RDA)	Drinking water (if naturally fluoride containing or fluoridated), tea, seafood	Fluorosis: discoloration of teeth
Selenium (no U.S. RDA)	Seafood, meat, grains	Digestive system disorders
Chromium (no U.S. RDA)	Meats, unrefined foods, fats, vegetable oils	Unknown as a nutrition disorder. Occupational exposures damage skin and kidneys
Molybdenum, Manganese (no U.S. RDA)	Molybdenum: legumes, cereals, organ meats. Manganese: widely distributed in foods	Molybdenum: enzyme inhibition. Manganese: poisoning, nervous system disorders
Cobalt (no U.S. RDA)	Meats, milk, and milk products	Unknown as a nutritional disorder

Water level in the body is maintained primarily by drinking fluids, but solid foods also contribute to water replenishment. Many foods — fruits, vegetables, and meats — contain large amounts of water. Even seemingly dry foods such as bread contain some water. Solid foods add water in another way — they contribute metabolic water, one of the by-products of their breakdown to energy sources.

Most water loss occurs through urination, while small quantities are lost in feces and in exhaled air from the lungs. Insensible perspiration (that which is not visible) accounts for a considerable amount of water loss. Since exercise and hot humid weather increase sweating, more water must be consumed during these times. Exercise in hot weather and water replacement guidelines were discussed in Chapter 4.

THE REDUCTION EQUATION: EXERCISE + SENSIBLE EATING = FAT CONTROL

Exercise is an important component for reducing body weight (specifically fat weight) while sparing or enhancing muscle tissue. Exercise uses calories, stimulates metabolism, and brings appetite in line with energy expenditure. On the other hand, dieting without exercise produces diminishing returns because metabolism slows down as caloric needs decrease. After a few weeks of dieting, the body goes into a survival mode and adapts to the reduced caloric intake. The diet becomes less effective, and continued weight loss is more difficult to accomplish. Eventually, the diet will end, some or all of the old eating patterns will be reestablished, and the lost weight will be regained. If dieting becomes cyclical, each attempt at losing weight may take longer, but the lost weight may be regained quicker, and

the likelihood that additional weight will be gained increases. Very-low calorie diets should be avoided. Without supplementation, it is impossible to receive the required nutrients, and the effects of low caloric intake on metabolism is devastating.

THE EFFECTS OF EXERCISE ON WEIGHT CONTROL

The often neglected factor in a weight loss attempt is exercise. Exercise and diet are not mutually exclusive. They are complementary in that each has a unique contribution to make to weight loss. The role of exercise was addressed in 1985 at an international meeting on obesity. The unanimous consensus of the experts was that "if you are about to start a weight reduction program or if you are trying to maintain your present weight, success or failure can depend on whether or not you exercise."

Exercise Burns Calories

The American College of Sports Medicine (ACSM) suggests that the minimal threshold of exercise for weight loss is 300 Kcals per exercise session performed at least three times a week or 200 Kcals per session performed at least four times a week.[8] These are minimum guidelines. You can turn to Tables 3.2, 3.4, and 3.5 in Chapter 3 because these contain the data that walkers and joggers can use to calculate the number of calories expended for a particular body weight at a specific speed for a given amount of time.

The Kcals burned during recovery from exercise contribute marginally to weight loss. The body does not shut off completely after exercise; it recovers gradually. Extra Kcals are burned during this period until metabolism returns to normal resting level. A rule of thumb is that 15 Kcals are burned in recovery for every 100 Kcals burned during exercise.[9] If 400 Kcals are used during exercise, an extra 60 Kcals will be used during the recovery period. Exercising at this level five days a week will result in approximately 4½ pounds lost in one year from the Kcals burned in recovery from exercise. This is illustrated by the following:

60 Kcals × 5 days = 300 Kcals/wk × 52 wks

$$= \frac{15,600 \ \text{Kcals/yr}}{3,500 \ \text{Kcals}}$$

$$= 4.45 \ \text{lbs}$$

Admittedly, this amount is not much, but it is a bonus that supplements the Kcals lost directly through exercise.

Exercise and Appetite: Eat More, Weigh Less

The results of animal and human studies during the past 35 years have been equivocal and confusing regarding the effect of exercise on appetite. The data have shown that exercise may decrease, increase, or have no effect upon food intake. Most studies have indicated that people either continued to eat the same amount or increased their food intake when they began exercising and were allowed to eat freely.

P. D. Wood investigated the effect of a year of jogging on previously sedentary middle-aged males.[10] The subjects were encouraged not to reduce their food intake or to attempt to lose weight during the course of the study. At the end of one year, the men who ran the most miles lost the most fat. The more miles they ran, the more they increased their food intake. Those who jogged the most miles (up to 25 miles per week) lost the most fat and the most weight and had the greatest increase in food

intake. Many studies have shown that active people consume more Kcals and are leaner than inactive people.

Two studies at St. Luke's Hospital in New York showed that the effect of exercise on the appetite is regulated to some extent by the degree of obesity at the start of the program.[11] Fifty-seven days of moderate treadmill exercise resulted in a 15-pound weight loss by obese female subjects. The women's caloric intake during exercise compared to the pre-exercise period was essentially unchanged. This study was repeated with women who were close to ideal weight according to insurance company charts. The results were very different. Moderate treadmill exercise produced an immediate surge in appetite, and the women maintained their "ideal body weight."

Exercise Stimulates Metabolism

Approximately 60% to 75% of the energy liberated from food is expended to maintain the essential functions of the body.[12] The energy to accomplish these functions is the basal metabolic rate (BMR) — the minimum amount of energy that the body expends to sustain life while at complete rest. The BMR is measured at least 12 hours since the last meal, after 8 hours of sleep, and in a thermally neutral environment (at a comfortable room temperature). Since these conditions are difficult to satisfy, they are often approximated, so that the BMR is estimated by the resting metabolic rate (RMR). The RMR requires that measurements be taken three to four hours after the last meal, following a 30-minute rest period in a thermally comfortable environment on a day in which the subject has not participated in vigorous physical activity.

Because of less muscle and more fat, the RMR of females is five to 10 percent lower than males and 15 percent lower than that of very muscular males. Males who are over-weight primarily because of heavy musculature have higher RMRs and respond more readily to exercise/diet approaches to weight loss than overweight men whose excess weight is primarily fat.[13] The energy needed to sustain the RMR constitutes a significant amount of the total number of daily calories expended by the average adult. Then, from a weight-management perspective, it is advantageous to preserve or enhance the RMR and to do nothing to reduce it. Exercise fits the bill very nicely.

A persistent misconception regarding exercise is that it does not burn enough Kcals to make the effort worthwhile. Actually, consistent participation in aerobic exercise (walking, jogging, cycling, rowing, aerobic dance, etc.) will burn substantial amounts of Kcals. Anaerobic activities such as weight training do not burn many Kcals during the workout, but they build the muscle tissue that will require more Kcals later on. Muscle-building activities are an investment in future weight control. In the long run, the increase in muscle mass increases metabolism so that the body's Kcal requirements increase even at rest. This is why activities for both cardiorespiratory development and muscular development are suggested for weight loss or weight maintenance or for any well-rounded physical fitness program.

In the past, the decline in RMR was presumed to be a natural aspect of aging. But age per se has relatively little effect. It seems that the acquired changes accompanying aging are primarily responsible for the decline in RMR. Muscle tissue uses more oxygen and more calories than fat during rest or physical activity. Authorities estimate that we lose 3% to 5% of our active protoplasm (mostly muscle tissue) each decade after 25 years of age. This loss is directly attributed to physical inactivity as we age and results in the all to common negative changes that are seen in body composition.

Physical activity is the key to weight management because it uses calories and accelerates metabolism. It also prevents or attenuates the weight-loss plateau that the majority of dieters experience. This plateau represents a period of time when weight loss decelerates substantially or stops temporarily.[14]

Lack of exercise has a negative effect on body composition (the amount of lean vs. fat tissues). For example, young and middle-aged subjects who were within plus or minus 5 percent of their ideal weight as determined by height, weight, and frame size charts illustrated the body composition changes that occur with age and physical inactivity. Although both groups were within the ideal range for weight, the middle-aged subjects had twice as much body fat as the young subjects. These data show quite well that lost muscle weight that is replaced by a gain in fat weight produces negative changes in body composition even in the absence of weight gain. Since fat is less dense than muscle, it occupies more room in the body; hence, the change in the configuration of the body. Table 7.8 illustrates some of the changes in the body composition that occur as American age. The examples are hypothetical, but they are based upon fact.

Subject 1 typifies the inactive person who maintains his body weight while aging but experiences a change in body composition. His bathroom scales provide no clues regarding the change, but the mirror and the fit of his clothes do. This man must hold a tight rein on appetite because his resting caloric requirements have diminished. Subject 2 is inactive and chooses to lose weight with age to keep from becoming fatter — rare in our society. He loses one quarter to one half a pound per year after age 30. This individual had lost muscle tissue and has reduced his body weight. His body composition has changed as a result — he is smaller all over. Because of the decline in

Table 7.8 Effects of Physical Inactivity on Body Composition

Subject	Body Weight at Age 20 (lb)	Body Weight at Age 60 (lb)	Activity Level	Lean Tissue*	Fat	Body Composition
1	150	150	Inactive	Lost 12%–20%	Gain	Changed
2	150	135	Inactive	Lost 12%–20%	No gain	Changed
3	150	165	Inactive	Lost 12%–20%	Gain	Changed
4	150	150	Active	No Loss	No gain	Unchanged

*The lean tissue values in the table apply to males, but the same trend is evident to a lesser degree in females because women have less lean tissue to lose.

Source: Adapted from M. Williams, *Nutrition for Fitness and Sport*, Dubuque, Iowa: Wm. C. Brown. Publishers, 1992.

metabolism from the loss of muscle along with a lower body weight, which diminishes the caloric cost of any weight-bearing movement, this individual must eat progressively less as the years pass to prevent a gain in fat tissue. Hunger would be a constant companion with this strategy. Subject 3 is probably most representative of the typical American who gains both fat and total weight with age. Subject 4 is physically active throughout life. He has little muscle loss and no gain in fat weight. Many examples of this modern-day phenomenon continue to jog, cycle, swim, and so on. Programs that build and maintain muscle tissue preserve the RMR and perpetuate a youthful body composition.

THE EFFECTS OF DIET ON WEIGHT CONTROL

Weight loss attempts in the United States have emphasized dietary restriction with continued sedentary living.[15] This combination has led to consistent failure. Weight loss with this method is temporary, and the majority of these weight watchers lose and gain weight many times during their lives. The eating patterns established during the diet period are short-lived.

Americans have been and continue to be obsessed with losing weight. At any given time, about 40% of women and 25% of men are attempting to lose weight for reasons of physical appearance or health.[16] Unfortunately, 90% to 95% of all dieters regain all or most of the weight that they lost within five years.[17] Eatless approaches to weight loss and permanent weight control have not worked and probably never will. It is notable that people repeatedly utilize weight-loss strategies that have failed them in the past. New attempts may feature new "diets," but calorie restriction remains the method of choice. It is time to forget dieting as an effective weight-loss technique. The appropriate nutritional approach emphasizes sensible modifications in eating behavior that can be followed for a lifetime, not for just a few weeks or a few months. This means a nutritional approach that emphasizes a low-fat, high complex carbohydrate style of eating. This combined with sensible, progressive, and consistent exercise for a lifetime should produce the permanent weight loss and control that people want.

Metabolism is adversely affected by calorie restriction. In its quest for homestasis (the tendency to maintain a constancy of internal conditions), the body adapts to the reduced-calorie intake by lowering the metabolic rate. This effort to economize in response to less food intake is a survival mechanism that protects people during lean times. Because the body learns to get by with less, the difference between calories eaten and calories needed narrows. This defense mechanism makes it possible for prisoners of war to survive internment in concentration camps. This same defense mechanism is operative in individuals who voluntarily reduce their food intake with the same result: a drop in RMR. As the RMR decreases, so too does the effectiveness of dieting. Regular vigorous exercise has the opposite effect: it accelerates the metabolic processes and increases body temperature during and after physical activity. The RMR may remain elevated for some time after exercise. Under exercise conditions, the body is spending Kcals rather than hoarding them.

Metabolism represents the body's production of heat. Exercise increases heat production, oxygen demand, and calories used. On the other hand, dieting without exercise reduces metabolic heat production and consequently the number of calories burned. Some studies have shown that several weeks of a very low calorie diet (less than 800 Kcals/day) resulted in a drop of heat production to 80% of the pre-diet level. This is counterproductive because weight loss under this procedure becomes more difficult. As the number of calories needed decreases, the difference between those needed and those consumed becomes smaller. The more restrictive the diet, the greater the loss of lean tissue and metabolic heat production.

Weight Cycling

Repeated weight loss and regain is referred to as weight cycling (also known as cycle dieting or yo-yo dieting). Cycle dieting may have significant negative effects on one's health and the practice may increase the difficulty of remaining at a desirable weight. The most serious consequences of cycle dieting are: (1) it increases the probability of all-cause mortality,[18] and (2) it increases the risk of dying from cardiovascular disease.[19]

The increased risk of developing cardiovascular disease has prompted researchers to conclude that it is probably better to remain a little overweight than to lose and regain the same 15 pounds over and over again.[20] Men who lost and regained 20 to 30 pounds during a given two-year period were at twice the risk of dying from cardiovascular disease than those whose weight remained reasonably constant. Women were at 1½ times the risk of dying from cardiovascular disease if they lost and regained 15 to 20 pounds during a two-year period. Two other long-term studies with thousands of subjects (the Multiple Risk Factor Intervention Trial and the Harvard Alumni Study) produced similar results.

The message is clear for those who need to lose weight: do it right the first time and commit to keeping the weight off. Cycle dieters, especially those with the greatest fluctuations, have the greatest risk.[21]

Waist-Hip Ratio (WHR)

Obesity increases the risk of premature morbidity (the sick rate in a population) and mortality (the death rate in a population), but the distribution of fat is as important as the amount of fat that is deposited. Fat that is regionally distributed in the abdomen, back, and chest (male pattern or android obesity) increases the risk of heart attack, stroke, Type II diabetes, and some forms of cancer.[22] As few as 10 to 15 pounds stored in this manner increases the risk. Fat stored in the hips, buttocks, and thighs (female pattern or gynoid obesity) is not as risky.

The pattern of fat deposition can be determined by calculating the waist/hip ratio (WHR). Ideally, the hips should be larger than the waist. Use a flexible tape to measure the circumference of your waist at the height of the navel. Then measure your hips at their largest circumference and divide the waist measurement by the hip measurement. The value obtained can be interpreted as follows:

1. Females — if the WHR is .8 or greater, the risk is higher than normal

2. Males — if the WHR is 1.0 or greater, the risk is higher than normal

Zuti and Golding investigated the relationship between exercise, diet, and weight loss.[23] They analyzed the effects of three different strategies upon the quantity and quality of weight loss. Each strategy was designed to elicit a loss of one pound per week. The subjects were overweight women 25 to 45 years of age. A summary of the results of the study appears in Table 7.9

The diet-only group reduced food intake by 500 Kcals per day and did not exercise. The exercise-only group did not diet but increased their physical activity by 500 Kcals per day. The diet-and-exercise group reduced their caloric intake by 250 Kcals per day while increasing their caloric expenditure by the same amount. The aim of all three strategies was to lose one pound per week (500 Kcals × 7 days = 3,500 Kcals), and this objective was essentially accomplished by all three groups.

But the significant outcome of this study was that 21 percent of the total loss experienced by the diet-only group was in the form of lean tissue. This occurred despite a nutritionally sound diet of modest calorie restriction. The other two groups lost fat (the true goal of weight-loss programs) and gained rather than lost lean tissue.

The results of this study have been corroborated by several other investigators, all of whom indicated that lean tissue is lost when diet restriction is not accompanied by exercise. The studies reinforced the need for including both sensible exercise and dietary modifications in a weight-loss program. The integrity of the muscular system can only be protected by participation in regular and systematic exercise and this benefit occurs whether or not one is dieting.

Some obese people seem to be diet resistant; that is, their weight remains stable even when they are following a low-calorie diet. This irony has been variously blamed upon an underactive thyroid, a slow metabolism, or a hereditary tendency toward obesity. A number of studies have shown that the actual reason for the majority of these cases is that these subjects tend to underreport their caloric intake and overestimate their physical activity. This dilemma was examined in a well-controlled study.[24] The researchers found that their diet-resistant subjects underestimated their food intake by 47 percent and overestimated their physical activity by 51 percent. The subjects perceived that their obesity was caused by

Table 7.9 Summary — Zuti/Golding Study

Weight Loss Strategy	Fat Tissue Loss (lb)	Lean Tissue Loss (lb)	Total Weight Loss (lb)
Diet only	− 9.3	−2.4	−11.7
Exercise only	−12.6	+2.0	−10.6
Diet and exercise	−13.0	+1.0	−12.0

genetic and metabolic factors rather than errors of judgment regarding caloric consumption and energy expenditure.

The American College of Sports Medicine (ACSM) produced a position paper entitled "Proper and Improper Weight Loss Programs." In it, the organization provided sensible guidelines, and with some minor modifications as identified by statements in parentheses below, are still appropriate today. Some of the important concepts addressed by ACSM include the following:*

1. A diet should provide at least 1200 Kcals/day to increase the likelihood of obtaining the necessary nutrients for the maintenance of good health. Diets that are calorically more restrictive are undesirable and potentially dangerous.

2. Food choices should be nutritionally balanced, palatable, and acceptable to the dieter.

3. Weight loss goals should be moderate — no more than 2 pounds per week. (Today there is support for limiting weight loss to 1½ pounds per week.)

4. Behavior modification techniques should be employed in conjunction with dietary modification and exercise to form a well-rounded approach to weight reduction.

5. An endurance type exercise program is a must. The minimum amount of exercise recommended for weight loss includes participation 20 to 30 minutes per day, 3 times per week, at 60% of the maximum heart rate. (If you expend 300 Kcals per exercise session you can exercise 3 times per week).

6. The dietary modifications and exercise program should be sustainable for a lifetime.

---

* American College of Sports Medicine. "Proper and Improper Weight Loss Programs," Medicine and Science in Sports and Exercise, 15 (1983): IX.

WEIGHT GAIN FOR THE UNDERWEIGHT

The focus thus far has been on weight loss rather than weight gain, but the purposeful gain of weight represents a real problem for the underweight. What constitutes underweight? This question has not been satisfactorily answered. Actuarial statistics indicate that those who are significantly below the average in body weight have a higher expected mortality rate. Marked underweight may be indicative of underlying disease and is as much of a risk as obesity for early death.

Being underweight may pose as much of a cosmetic problem for an affected individual as obesity is for an obese individual. An effective weight-gain program should include regular participation in resistance exercise in conjunction with three well-balanced meals plus a couple of nutritious between-meal snacks. There are some commercial drinks that are useful for increasing caloric consumption. Protein supplementation is unnecessary and can be harmful if taken in excessive amounts. Despite Herculean efforts, many underweight people find it more difficult to gain a pound than it is for the obese to lose one. Very lean people should not attempt to gain weight by increasing the fat content of their diet. This is an unhealthy eating pattern for anyone regardless of body weight.

The amount and type of weight gain should be closely monitored. It is desirable to gain muscle tissue without increasing fat stores. Overeating without exercise will not accomplish this objective, nor will it enhance physical appearance. Body fat should not be increased unless affected individuals are so thin that they may be in danger of dipping into essential fat, which is necessary for the life processes.

MEASURING OVERWEIGHT

Overweight is defined as excess weight for one's height. It is assessed by using a height/weight chart. If your weight falls above the acceptable range, you are overweight. This approach does not make allowances for body composition, it just provides information about weight status without considering the amount of fluid, fat, or muscle make-up of an individual. Two people of the same sex, same height and same weight could conceivably be very different in physical appearance because one may be carrying excess fat while the other is carrying substantial muscle tissue. Beside the difference in physical appearance, the risk of developing premature chronic disease is associated with excess fat not muscle.

Body Mass Index (BMI)

A method for assessing overweight that is becoming very popular with medical and nutrition researchers is the body mass index (BMI). Indeed, some authorities consider it to be the best available method for assessing excess poundage.[25] Its inherent limitation, since it is based on height and weight, is similar to that of the height/weight tables. Muscular people may fall into the overweight category without being overfat. The advantages of this method include: (1) the ease with which it can be determined, (2) the establishment of BMI categories that identify weight status, and (3) the identification of BMI levels that constitute a risk for cardiovascular disease.

Body mass index is calculated by dividing body weight in kilograms (kg) by height in meters (m) squared. But there is a simpler method that does not require conversion from the U.S. system of measurement to the metric equivalents and it loses very little accuracy in

the process. For the sake of simplicity we will use the following formula:

$$BMI = \frac{Body\ wt.\ (lbs)\ \times\ 700}{Ht.\ (in.)^2}$$

If a female weighs 158 lbs. and is 5'3" tall, her BMI would be calculated as follows:

1. Convert height in feet and inches to inches
   5'3" is equal to 63"

2. Square height in inches $(63)^2 = 3969$

3. $BMI = \dfrac{158 \times 700}{3969}$

   $= \dfrac{110600}{3969}$

   $= 27.9$

Body mass index standards have been suggested by the American College of Sports Medicine (ACSM).[26] BMIs of 21 to 23 are considered desirable for women; 22 to 24 are desirable for men. The risk of cardiovascular disease increases substantially when BMIs equal or surpass 27.3 for women and 27.8 for men. Table 7.10 gives the body weight classification for various BMI values for men and women. The female in our example, with a BMI of 27.9 has an increased risk for a heart attack according to ACSM guidelines and is in the overweight category according to Table 7.10.

MEASURING BODY COMPOSITION

Body composition assessment requires the separation and quantification of lean tissue from fat. Many indirect methods for measuring this component have been developed but we will focus on just one — skinfold measurements.

Table 7.10   Weight Classification by BMI

BMI (males)	BMI (females)	Classification
*<20.7	*<19.1	Underweight
20.7–26.4	19.2–25.8	Acceptable Weight
26.5–27.8	25.9–27.3	Marginal overweight
27.9–31.1	27.4–32.2	Overweight
31.2–45.4	32.3–44.8	Severe overweight
**>45.4	**>44.8	Morbid Obesity

*< less than
**> greater than

Adapted from E. N. Whitney and S. R. Rolfes, *Understanding Nutrition, St. Paul: West Publishing Co., 1993.*

Lean tissue includes all tissue exclusive of fat: muscle, bones, organs, fluid, and so on. Fat includes both essential and storage fat. Essential fat, found in the bone marrow, organs, muscles, intestines, and central nervous system, is indispensable to normal physiological functioning. The amount of essential fat in the male body is equal to approximately 3% to 5% of the total body weight. The amount of essential fat in the female body is equal to about 11% to 14% of the total body weight. The disparity in the amount of essential fat between the sexes is probably because of sex-specific essential fat stored in a female's breast, pelvic area, and thighs. Essential fat constitutes a lower limit beyond which fat loss is undesirable and unhealthy because of the possibility of impaired normal physiological and biological functioning from such loss.

Storage fat is found in adipose tissue. For most Americans, this represents a substantial energy reserve. Adipose tissue is found subcutaneously (under the skin) and around the organs, where it acts as a buffer against physical trauma. It is desirable to reduce excess storage fat for health and aesthetic reasons. Reasonable goals for total body fat (essential plus storage fat) differ for both sexes. Excellent values for males and females are 12 percent

and 18 percent, respectively. Males are overfat when 23% to 25% of their weight is in the form of fat; females are overfat when 32% or more of their weight is in the form of fat.

Skinfold measurement in becoming more commonplace since several low cost calipers have made their way into the marketplace. In skilled hands, some of them correlate quite well (.90) with the more expensive brands found in most exercise physiology labs. The rationale for this technique is based on the fact that approximately fifty percent of the body's fat is located directly beneath the skin, therefore the skinfold, which is a double layer of skin and the underlying fat, may be measured with a caliper. In this text, the Jackson and Pollock generalized tables for age and sex are used to convert skinfold measurement (in millimeters) to percent fat. See Tables 7.11 and 7.12.

To become proficient, one must practice measuring the different sites for all ages and both sexes. The method can be standardized by observing the following suggestions:

1. Mark each site according to the directions given in Figures 7.5 through 7.9.

2. Take two measurements at each site, unless there is a difference of more than one millimeter between the two; if there is, take a

Table 7.11   Percent Fat Estimates For Men*

Sum of Skinfolds (mm)	Age to the Last Year								
	Under 22	23 to 27	28 to 32	33 to 37	38 to 42	43 to 47	48 to 52	53 to 57	Over 57
8– 10	1.3	1.8	2.3	2.9	3.4	3.9	4.5	5.0	5.5
11– 13	2.2	2.8	3.3	3.9	4.4	4.9	5.5	6.0	6.5
14– 16	3.2	3.8	4.3	4.8	5.4	5.9	6.4	7.0	7.5
17– 19	4.2	4.7	5.3	5.8	6.3	6.9	7.4	8.0	8.5
20– 22	5.1	5.7	6.2	6.8	7.3	7.9	8.4	8.9	9.5
23– 25	6.1	6.6	7.2	7.7	8.3	8.8	9.4	9.9	10.5
26– 28	7.0	7.6	8.1	8.7	9.2	9.8	10.3	10.9	11.4
29– 31	8.0	8.5	9.1	9.6	10.2	10.7	11.3	11.8	12.4
32– 34	8.9	9.4	10.0	10.5	11.5	11.6	12.2	12.8	13.3
35– 37	9.8	10.4	10.9	11.5	12.0	12.6	13.1	13.7	14.3
38– 40	10.7	11.3	11.8	12.4	12.9	13.5	14.1	14.6	15.2
41– 43	11.6	12.2	12.7	13.3	13.8	14.4	15.0	15.5	16.1
44– 46	12.5	13.1	13.6	14.2	14.7	15.3	15.9	16.4	17.0
47– 49	13.4	13.9	14.5	15.1	15.6	16.2	16.8	17.3	17.9
50– 52	14.3	14.8	15.4	15.9	16.5	17.1	17.6	18.2	18.8
53– 55	15.1	15.7	16.2	16.8	17.4	17.9	18.5	19.1	19.7
56– 58	16.0	16.5	17.1	17.7	18.2	18.8	19.4	20.0	20.5
59– 61	16.9	17.4	17.9	18.5	19.1	19.7	20.2	20.8	21.4
62– 64	17.6	18.2	18.8	19.4	19.9	20.5	21.1	21.7	22.2
65– 67	18.5	19.0	19.6	20.2	20.8	21.3	21.9	22.5	23.1
68– 70	19.3	19.9	20.4	21.0	21.6	22.2	22.7	23.3	23.9
71– 73	20.1	20.7	21.2	21.8	22.4	23.0	23.6	24.1	24.7
74– 76	20.9	21.5	22.0	22.6	23.2	23.8	24.4	25.0	25.5
77– 79	21.7	22.2	22.8	23.4	24.0	24.6	25.2	25.8	26.3
80– 82	22.4	23.0	23.6	24.2	24.8	25.4	25.9	26.5	27.1
83– 85	23.2	23.8	24.4	25.0	25.5	26.1	26.7	27.3	27.9
86– 88	24.0	24.5	25.1	25.7	26.3	26.9	27.5	28.1	28.7
89– 91	24.7	25.3	25.9	26.5	27.1	27.6	28.2	28.8	29.4
92– 94	25.4	26.0	26.6	27.2	27.8	28.4	29.0	29.6	30.2
95– 97	26.1	26.7	27.3	27.9	28.5	29.1	29.7	30.3	30.9
98–100	26.9	27.4	28.0	28.6	29.2	29.8	30.4	31.0	31.6
101–103	27.5	28.1	28.7	29.3	29.9	30.5	31.1	31.7	32.3
104–106	28.2	28.8	29.4	30.0	30.6	31.2	31.8	32.4	33.0
107–109	28.9	29.5	30.1	30.7	31.3	31.9	32.5	33.1	33.7
110–112	29.6	30.2	30.8	31.4	32.0	32.6	33.2	33.8	34.4
113–115	30.2	30.8	31.4	32.0	32.6	33.2	33.8	34.5	35.1
116–118	30.9	31.5	32.1	32.7	33.3	33.9	34.5	35.1	35.7
119–121	31.5	32.1	32.7	33.3	33.9	34.5	35.1	35.7	36.4
122–124	32.1	32.7	33.3	33.9	34.5	35.1	35.8	36.4	37.0
125–127	32.7	33.3	33.9	34.5	35.1	35.8	36.4	37.0	37.6

*Sum of chest, abdominal, and thigh skinfolds.

From Jackson, A. S. and M. L. Pollock. (May, 1985) "Practical Assessment of Body Composition." *The Physician and Sportsmedicine* 13, No. 5, pp. 76-90. Reprinted by permission.

Table 7.12   Percent Fat Estimates For Women*

Sum of Skinfolds (mm)	Age to the Last Year								
	Under 22	23 to 27	28 to 32	33 to 37	38 to 42	43 to 47	48 to 52	53 to 57	Over 57
23– 25	9.7	9.9	10.2	10.4	10.7	10.9	11.2	11.4	11.7
26– 28	11.0	11.2	11.5	11.7	12.0	12.3	12.5	12.7	13.0
29– 31	12.3	12.5	12.8	13.0	13.3	13.5	13.8	14.0	14.3
32– 34	13.6	13.8	14.0	14.3	14.5	14.8	15.0	15.3	15.5
35– 37	14.8	15.0	15.3	15.5	15.8	16.0	16.3	16.5	16.8
38– 40	16.0	16.3	16.5	16.7	17.0	17.2	17.5	17.7	18.0
41– 43	17.2	17.4	17.7	17.9	18.2	18.4	18.7	18.9	19.2
44– 46	18.3	18.6	18.8	19.1	19.3	19.6	19.8	20.1	20.3
47– 49	19.5	19.7	20.0	20.2	20.5	20.7	21.0	21.2	21.5
50– 52	20.6	20.8	21.1	21.3	21.6	21.8	22.1	22.3	22.6
53– 55	21.7	21.9	22.1	22.4	22.6	22.9	23.1	23.4	23.6
56– 58	22.7	23.0	23.2	23.4	23.7	23.9	24.2	24.4	24.7
59– 61	23.7	24.0	24.2	24.5	24.7	25.0	25.2	25.5	25.7
62– 64	24.7	25.0	25.2	25.5	25.7	26.0	26.2	26.4	26.7
65– 67	25.7	25.9	26.2	26.4	26.7	26.9	27.2	27.4	27.7
68– 70	26.6	26.9	27.1	27.4	27.6	27.9	28.1	28.4	28.6
71– 73	27.5	27.8	28.0	28.3	28.5	28.8	29.0	29.3	29.5
74– 76	28.4	28.8	28.9	29.2	29.4	29.7	29.9	30.2	30.4
77– 79	29.3	29.5	29.8	30.0	30.3	30.5	30.8	31.0	31.3
80– 82	30.1	30.4	30.6	30.9	31.1	31.4	31.6	31.9	32.1
83– 85	30.9	31.2	31.4	31.7	31.9	32.2	32.4	32.7	32.9
86– 88	31.7	32.0	32.2	32.5	32.7	32.9	33.2	33.4	33.7
89– 91	32.5	32.7	33.0	33.2	33.5	33.7	33.9	34.2	34.4
92– 94	33.2	33.4	33.7	33.9	34.2	34.4	34.7	34.9	35.2
95– 97	33.9	34.1	34.4	34.6	34.9	35.1	35.4	35.6	35.9
98–100	34.6	34.8	35.1	35.3	35.5	35.8	36.0	36.3	36.5
101–103	35.3	35.4	35.7	35.9	36.2	36.4	36.7	36.9	37.2
104–106	35.8	36.1	36.3	36.6	36.8	37.1	37.3	37.5	37.8
107–109	36.4	36.7	36.9	37.1	37.4	37.6	37.9	38.1	38.4
110–112	37.0	37.2	37.5	37.7	38.0	38.2	38.5	38.7	38.9
113–115	37.5	37.8	38.0	38.2	38.5	38.7	39.0	39.2	39.5
116–118	38.0	38.3	38.5	38.8	39.0	39.3	39.5	39.7	40.0
119–121	38.5	38.7	39.0	39.2	39.5	39.7	40.0	40.2	40.5
122–124	39.0	39.2	39.4	39.7	39.9	40.2	40.4	40.7	40.9
125–127	39.4	39.6	39.9	40.0	40.4	40.6	40.9	41.1	41.4
128–130	39.8	40.0	40.3	40.5	40.8	41.0	41.3	41.5	41.8

*Sum of triceps, suprailium, and thigh skinfolds..

From Jackson, A. S. and M. L. Pollock (May, 1985) "Practical Assessment of Body Composition," *The Physician and Sportsmedicine* 13, No. 5: pp. 76–90. Reprinted by permission.

third measurement and average the two closest readings.

3. The calipers should be applied about one quarter to one half of an inch below the fingers. This allows the calipers rather than the fingers to compress the skinfold.

4. The calipers should maintain contact with the skinfold for two to five seconds so that the reading can stabilize.

SKINFOLD MEASUREMENT SITES

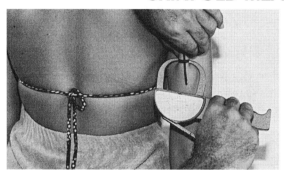

Figure 7.5 Triceps Skinfold. Take a vertical fold on the midline of the upper arm over the triceps halfway between the acromion and olecranon processes (tip of shoulder to tip of elbow). The arm should be extended and relaxed when the measurement is taken.

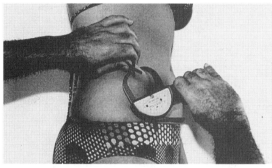

Figure 7.6 Suprailium Skinfold. Take a diagonal fold above the crest of the ilium directly below the mid-axilla (armpit).

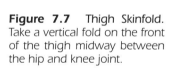

Figure 7.7 Thigh Skinfold. Take a vertical fold on the front of the thigh midway between the hip and knee joint.

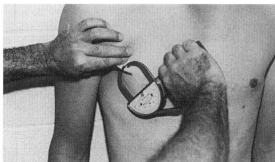

Figure 7.8 Chest Skinfold. Take a diagonal fold one-half the distance between the anterior axillary line and nipple.

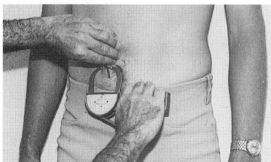

Figure 7.9 Abdominal Skinfold. Take a vertical fold about 3/8 inch from the navel.

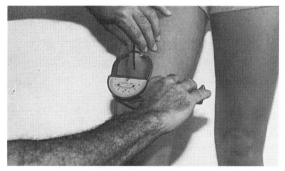

Summary

- Metabolism is the sum total of chemical reactions whereby the energy liberated from food is made available to the body. It consists of two processes — anabolism and catabolism.

- The Food Guide Pyramid has replaced the basic four food group.

- The new food labels mandated by the federal government for processed food will help consumers to make more informed decisions regarding food choices.

- Carbohydrates consist of simple sugars and starches.

- Sugar causes tooth decay but it is not an independent risk factor for chronic diseases except in rare cases.

- There are two types of dietary fiber — soluble and insoluble. These are indigestible polysaccharides that are beneficial to health.

- Carbohydrates yield 4 Kcals/gram.

- Fats are energy dense yielding 9 Kcals/gram.

- Saturated fats come from animal flesh, dairy products, and tropical oils. These raise serum cholesterol levels.

- Unsaturated fats come from plants and should constitute the majority of the fat that we consume.

- Dietary fat should be less than 30% of the total calories.

- Trans fatty acids may be as harmful as saturated fats.

- Protein intake should be about 12% of the total calories.

- Adults need .8 of a gram of protein per kg of body weight; endurance athletes may require twice this amount.

- The fat soluble vitamins are A, D, E, and K; the water soluble vitamins are C, and B complex.

- Antioxidant vitamins may play an important role in the prevention of cardiovascular disease and cancer.

- Minerals are inorganic substances that exist freely in nature.

- Exercise is an important component of weight management.

- Exercise burns calories and stimulates metabolism.

- Dieting decreases caloric intake, reduces metabolism and lean body tissue.

- Most dieters regain the lost weight within five years.

- Weight cycling increases the risk of cardiovascular disease.

- Android obesity increases the risk of heart attack, stroke, Type II diabetes, and some forms of cancer.

- Body mass index (BMI) is a good method for determining one's weight status.

- Males have less essential fat than females.

- Skinfold measurement techniques are inexpensive, quick, and effective for measuring percent body fat.

REFERENCES

1. "Database," *U.S. News and World Report*, 113, No. 23: (December 14, 1992), p. 12.

2. "Myth: Fruit Juice Concentration is a More Healthful Sweetener Than Sugar," *University of California at Berkeley Wellness Letter*, 9, Issue 2: (September, 1993), p. 8.

3. Dahl, L. J. "Sugars and Fats: The Tip of the Food Pyramid," *Cardi Sense*, IV, No. 2: (1994), p. 6.

4. "Fish Oil Capsules vs. Fish" *University of California at Berkeley Wellness Letter*, 10, Issue 9: (June, 1994) , p. 4.

5. "Margarine: Spare the Stick, Save the Child," *Harvard Heart Letter*, 3, No. 11: (July, 1993), p. 4.

6. Whitney, E. N. and Rolfes, S.R. *Understanding Nutrition*, St. Paul: West Publishing Co., 1993.

7. Liebman, B. "The Salt Shake Out," *Nutrition Action Health Letter*, 21, No. 2: (March, 1994), p. 1.

8. ACSM. "The Recommended Quantity and Quality of Exercise for Developing and Maintaining Cardiorespiratory and Muscular Fitness in Healthy Adults," *Medicine and Science in Sports*, 22: (1990) p. 265.

9. Nieman, D. C. *Fitness and Sports Medicine: An Introduction*, Palo Alto, CA: Bull Publishing, 1990.

10. Wood, P. D. et al. "Increased Exercise Level and Plasma Lipoprotein Concentrations: A One-year Randomized, Controlled Study in Sedentary Middle-Aged Men," *Metabolism*, 32: (1983), p. 31.

11. Wood, P. *California Diet and Exercise Program*, Mountain View, CA: Anderson World Books, 1983.

12. McArdle, W. D., Katch, F. I., and Katch, V. L. *Exercise Physiology*, Philadelphia: Lea and Febiger, 1991.

13. Pierre, C. "Maximizing Metabolism: Can Calorie Burning Be Increased?" *Environmental Nutrition*, 12: (February, 1989) , p. 1.

14. Seigel, A. J. "New Insights About Obesity and Exercise," *Your Patient and Fitness*, 2: (January/February 1989), p 12.

15. "Losing Weight: A New Attitude Emerges," *Harvard Heart Letter*, 4, No. 7: (March, 1994), 3 p. 1.

16. "Heavy News," *University of California at Berkeley Wellness Letter*, 10, Issue 5: (February, 1994), p. 2.

17. Wing, R.R. "Weight Cycling in Humans: A Review of the Literature," *Annals of Behavioral Medicine*, 14: (1992), p. 113.

18. Lissner, L. et al. "Variability of Body Weight and Health Outcomes in the Framingham Population," *New England Journal of Medicine*, 324: (1991), p. 1839.

19. Lissner, L., et al.

20. Lissner, L., et al.

21. Lissner, L., et al.

22. Lissner, L., et al.

23. Zuti, B. and Golding, L. "Comparing Diet and Exercise as Weight Reduction Tools," *The Physician and Sportsmedicine*, 4: (1976), p. 49.

24. Lichtman, S. W. et al. "Discrepancy Between Self-Reported and Actual Caloric Intake and Exercise in Obese Subjects," *New England Journal of Medicine*, 327: (1992), p. 1893.

25. "Heavy News."

26. ACSM. *Guidelines for Exercise Testing and Prescription*, Philadelphia: Lea and Febiger, 1991.

Prevention and Treatment of Walking and Jogging Injuries

Terms

- Amenorrhea
- Concentric muscle contraction
- Eccentric muscle contraction
- Estrogen
- Inflammation
- Menstruation
- Orthotic
- R-I-C-E principle

This chapter focuses on injuries that may occur to walkers and joggers. All exercise participants will incur an injury or two if they exercise long enough. Fortunately, most are minor and respond to minimal level treatment. The aim of this chapter is to reinforce the importance of prevention of injuries, but also to present some injuries common to walking and jogging in order to acquaint you with recognizable symptoms and effective treatments. Recognizing the symptoms is the first step in treating the injury and it is important for treatment to begin as soon as possible after an injury has occurred.

PRINCIPLES OF INJURY PREVENTION

The often-heard adage, "an ounce of prevention is worth a pound of cure" is applicable when one embarks upon a walking or jogging program. It continues to be appropriate advice even for seasoned participants because after an injury-free period some of them become complacent and disregard the principles which have contributed to the avoidance of injury. The best way to deal with injuries is to prevent their occurrence. Previous chapters have focused upon the principles of training which are designed to promote aerobic fitness with maximum safety, some of these are:

1. Contain your enthusiasm. Enthusiasm is necessary for success, but too much may lead to overexertion and injury.

Increasing the distance or decreasing the time required to cover a given distance should occur slowly and progressively.

2. Those with multiple risks or those over 45 years of age should obtain clearance for jogging by a physician.

3. The program should be individualized to meet the exerciser's aims and objectives.

4. The exercise intensity of each workout should not exceed 85% of maximal heart rate.

5. The duration of each workout should be within the 20 to 30 minute range in the early stages of the program and be lengthened as fitness improves.

6. In the beginning, walk or jog every other day and increase the frequency to a level which is consistent with physical improvement and program objectives.

7. Wear quality walking and jogging shoes.

8. Adjust the intensity and duration of the workout according to the environmental conditions.

9. Hydrate fully prior to the workout, continue to drink liquid during and after the workout.

10. Follow sound warm-up and cool-down procedures.

11. Work to improve walking and jogging form.

12. Choose surfaces that are less likely to promote injuries.

► TREATING COMMON INJURIES

General Treatment — The R-I-C-E Principle

The R-I-C-E (Rest, Ice, Compression, and Elevation) will help to reduce the pain, swelling, and inflammation.[1]

1. **Rest:** Rest is advised if movement produces pain in the affected area.

2. **Ice:** Apply ice immediately for 15 to 20 minutes and repeat ice application every few hours. Do not apply ice for more than 20 minutes at a time. A convenient way to apply ice is to put crushed ice or ice cubes in a large size plastic freezer bag and place it on the injured area. As the ice melts, it will not leak.

3. **Compression:** Use an elastic bandage between icing to wrap the injured area. Do not keep the wrap on when you sleep and loosen it if the injured area begins to throb or change color.

4. **Elevation:** Elevating the injured area should help to keep the swelling down. Do this several times during the day.

Treatment of Selected Injuries

Achilles Tendon Injuries

The achilles tendon connects the calf muscle to the heel of the foot. Achilles tendonitis is a painful inflammation which is often accompanied by swelling. Jogging uphill, walking or jogging shoes with inflexible soles, and failure to maintain a stretching program are the three most frequent causes of achilles tendonitis. The symptoms include burning pain which usually appears early in the workout and then subsides until the exercise ends at which time the pain reappears and progressively worsens.

Treatment includes icing the tendon followed by gently stretching. Prevention involves daily stretching to increase calf flexibility and the use of quality walking or jogging shoes.[2] Preventive maintenance is important because the tendon may tear or rupture under stress. In the latter case, surgery becomes the only effective treatment, but either situation leads to a long period of inactivity.[3]

Blisters

Blisters are painful friction burns of a minor nature that result in fluid filled sacs of various sizes. Blisters may be prevented by wearing properly fitted shoes, clean socks, and employing the correct footstrike. Additionally, foot or talcum powder may be sprinkled inside socks and shoes to reduce friction.

Apply moleskin (toughskin) to those areas of the feet where there is a higher tendency to form blisters. "Hot spots" are reddened areas which will become blisters very quickly if preventive measures are not taken. Should a blister form, wash the area thoroughly with soap and water and apply a generous coat of iodine to it and the surrounding area. Then use a sterile needle to puncture the blister at its base and squeeze out the accumulated fluid. When this is completed apply an antiseptic mediation and a sterile dressing. Exercise may be continued after treatment by cutting a doughnut from foam rubber and taping it over the blister.

Chafing

Chafing usually occurs in areas where there is a high degree of friction. For example, people with large thighs that rub together will experience chaffing. This a minor but aggravating injury which can easily be prevented by applying a generous coat of vaseline to susceptible areas prior to the workout. Treatment for chafing is immediate cessation of walking and jogging with the onset of irritation and the application of an antiseptic lotion.

Chondromalacia Patella

Chondromalacia patella (*chondro* — cartilage; *malacia* —softening; patella — kneecap) is commonly referred to as "runner's knee." This describes a condition which occurs when the kneecap tracks laterally rather than vertically during flexion and extension of the leg. Typical symptoms include soreness around and under the kneecap particularly when jogging uphill or climbing stairs. The pain must be eliminated before jogging can be safely resumed. Treatment includes rest, application of ice, and aspirin every four hours for several weeks. Ice treatment should be discontinued after 24 to 36 hours and replaced with moist heat several times per day for as long as needed.

When pain abates, the jogger may begin progressive resistance exercises to strengthen the quadriceps group (large muscles in the front of the thigh) and a low intensity graduated jogging program. Preventive measures include (1) the use of orthotic devices (supports placed in jogging shoes to compensate for biomechanical problems). These are designed to prevent abnormal motions in the foot and lower leg during jogging, (2) avoidance of hard running surfaces such as concrete sidewalks, (3) abstaining from sloped or hilly terrain, and, (4) hold stair-climbing to a minimum.

Hamstring Injuries

The hamstrings are a group of muscles in the back of the thigh. The muscles in this group are subject to strains or tears.[4] There is usually a specific area of pain directly over the area of injury. Muscles strains usually occur within the belly or central part of the muscle. Severe strains usually occur in the tendon where the muscle originates or connects to the bones. Hamstring tears occur either high in the thigh next to the buttocks or down low just above the knee. When tears are on the inside of the thigh, they usually occur close to the groin.

Use the R-I-C-E principle in treating hamstring injuries. You should perform mild static stretching of the hamstrings as long as no pain occurs. Do not force the stretches because the injury may become aggravated.

Low Back Pain

Strains that cause the muscles to spasm constitute 90% of all low back pain. Strains may be attributed to many varied causes but those which commonly precipitate problems for walkers and joggers are: (1) weak abdominal muscles, (2) tight low back and hamstring muscles, (3) overuse — increasing the mileage too rapidly, and (4) faulty mechanics, particularly too much forward lean.

Preventive measures include daily stretching of the low back and hamstrings, strengthening of the abdominals, slowly increasing mileage, and improving faulty walking and jogging mechanics. Walking and jogging strengthen the muscles of the lower back; stretching exercises keep them from shortening. At the same time, the abdominal muscles need to be strengthened because they provide some support to the spinal column in holding up the weight of the torso. Treatment of low back pain includes rest, aspirin, and a firm mattress with a bed board.

Morton's Neuroma

Morton's Neuroma results in burning pain between the third and fourth toes usually as a result of repetitive trauma, such as that experienced by runners. Trauma is the primary cause and pain is the primary symptom. Pain is the result of scar tissue (fibrosis) impinging upon the sensory digital nerve, and may be constant or it might appear after walking or jogging on a hard surface. Narrow shoes, and particularly high-heeled shoes, should be avoided. Treatment may include the use of metatarsal bars or pads which are worn across the ball of the foot, shoes with a wide toebox, and local injection of a steroid preparation. Rest is suggested as long as the individual responds with pain to finger pressure at the site. If all of the above fail then surgery will be required. Prevention includes wearing walking, jogging and everyday shoes that are roomy in the toebox, well padded under the balls of the feet, and flexible. Walking and jogging on softer surfaces also helps.

Muscle Cramps

Muscle cramps are sudden, powerful, involuntary muscle contractions which produce considerable pain. Some cramps are recurrent, that is, they are characterized by repeated contractions and relaxation of the muscles, while others produce steady continuous contraction. Preventive measures include a gradual warm-up which includes stretching exercises. Overfatigue should be avoided.

Causes associated with muscle cramping are difficult to establish. Fatigue, depletion of both body fluids and minerals, and loss of muscle coordination have all been implicated to some extent.

Muscle cramps should not be massaged because there may be underlying blood vessel damage and internal bleeding. Vigorous massage in this case would aggravate the condition and promote additional damage. Treatment should include firm, consistent pressure at the site of the cramp. This should be followed by the application of ice and then the affected muscle should be stretched.

Muscle Soreness

Muscle soreness subsequent to walking and jogging is probably due to microscopic tears in muscle fibers and damage to muscle membranes.[5] This damage is partially responsible for the localized pain, tenderness and swelling experienced by exercisers 24 to 48 hours after the workout. Downhill running and walking have been implicated in delayed muscle soreness.[6] In downhill running, the leg muscles contract eccentrically, that is, they produce force as they lengthen. Running uphill produces the opposite effect as the muscles contract concentrically to provide the lift needed to negotiate the upgrade. To further expand upon this concept, when a weight is lifted, the muscles contract concentrically to produce the force needed to raise the weight against the force of gravity. When the weight is set down, the muscles contract eccentrically, lengthen, and produce the same amount of force to slow its descent. It is this portion of the movement that results in delayed muscle soreness. In a simple yet ingenious study, Newham and others had their subjects exercise by consistently stepping onto a box with one leg and stepping down with the other.[7] The step-up represented the concentric contraction and the step down was the eccentric contraction. The subjects experienced pain which peaked 48 hours after the exercise in the eccentrically exercised leg only.

The delayed soreness experienced with eccentric exercise is probably due to the recruitment of only a few muscle fibers which must produce great tension to perform the work. Untrained people experience greater delayed muscle soreness than trained people.

Delayed muscle soreness may be prevented by keeping the intensity, duration and frequency of exercise within one's ability level, by progressing slowly, by doing daily stretching exercises and by walking and jogging on a flat surface in the initial stages of training. As one becomes more fit, uphill and downhill walking and running should be carefully included in the routine. If soreness occurs, it should be treated with rest as well as stretching the affected muscles several times per day.

Plantar Fasciitis

Occasionally, low grade pain beneath the heel of one or both feet occurs. In mild cases, this pain can be felt during jogging, but more severe cases produce pain upon walking also.[8] The pain results from microscopic tears and inflammation of the connective tissue (planter fascia) beneath the heel. Treatment consists of cold therapy several times a day for the first few days, rest, anti-inflammatory drugs, heel pads, and possibly orthotic correction. Orthotics are supports which are placed in the walking and running shoes which are designed to correct the biomechanical problems which may have contributed to plantar fasciitis. Prevention involves well-fitted, well-cushioned walking and jogging shoes and a stretching program that includes stretching the calf and achilles tendon.

Shin Splints

Shin splints produce pain which radiates along the inner surface of the large bone of the lower leg. It is caused by running or walking on hard surfaces in improper shoes. It is most prevalent among unconditioned or novice exercisers who do too much too soon.[9] Jogging or walking in one direction on a banked track or banked road shoulder can also contribute to shin splints. Shin splints are the most common running injury.[10]

Pain associated with this injury manifests itself gradually. Initially, it occurs after the workout, but as training continues, it tends to show up during the workout. In severe cases, pain may accompany walking and stair climbing. Treatment includes rest, ice applications, wrapping or taping the shin, and placing heel lifts in the shoes.

These may be supplemented by the following exercises. The Toe Flexor exercise is accomplished by sitting in a chair with the bare feet approximately shoulder width apart. Place a towel on the floor in front of both feet allowing the toes to overlap the near edge of the towel. Repeatedly curl the toes in order to pull the towel toward you so that it ends up under the arch of the feet. The heels must be in contact with the floor at all times. You may place a weight, such as a book or can of vegetables, upon the towel to increase the resistance. The Toe Extensor exercise is the reverse of the Toe Flexor. By reversing the action of the toes you will push the towel away from you and return it to the original position. Keep your heels on the floor. For the Sandsweeper exercise sit on a chair with one bare foot on the lateral edge of a towel. Grasp the towel with the toes and pivot on the heel to the right to sweep the towel in that direction. Return the foot to the starting position and repeat until the towel has been moved completely to the right. Replace the towel to the original position and sweep to the left. Repeat with the other foot.

Shin splints are nagging, painful injuries that are best prevented rather than treated. Some preventive measures include wearing quality walking or jogging shoes, gradual adjustments to the rigors of training, avoidance of hard surfaces and hilly terrain, proper heel-toe strike, and daily use of the exercises previously described.

Stress Fractures

Stress fractures are tiny, often microscopic breaks in bones. Particularly affected are the bones of the feet and shins. The symptoms include one or all of the following: dull ache, local tenderness, and swelling. Pain also occurs when pressure is applied to the site of injury.

This is a classic injury of overuse. Exercisers who are logging too many miles, exercising too often, and on hard surfaces, are candidates for stress fractures. Surfaces that have little or no "give" or "resiliency" force the body to absorb

more of the shock.[11] This applies to joggers in particular because the shock of landing is high. Quality jogging shoes are a must, but they can only absorb a portion of the shock.

Women who are training heavily are susceptible to stress fractures particularly if they become lean enough to stop their menstrual cycle. When the menstrual cycle stops so does the production of estrogen (female sex hormone). Estrogen protects the bones from thinning out. A female runner who is amenorrheic (stoppage of the normal menstrual cycle) for a couple of years has lost a significant amount of bony tissue and this, in combination with vigorous training, leaves her vulnerable to stress fractures. The risk of stress fractures for women can be reduced by cutting back on mileage and by not becoming so lean as to interrupt the process of menstruation.

Rest is essential if a stress fracture has been diagnosed. Follow the advice of your physician regarding your return to physical activity. When you are cleared for exercise, you cannot pick up where you left off when you were injured. Start at a low level and gradually increase the duration, frequency, and lastly, the intensity of exercise. Be sure to stretch properly before and after exercise and select walking and jogging surfaces that have some give. Artificial surfaces (such as those found on football fields and running tracks), flat grassy surfaces that are free of holes (such as public parks and golf courses), and cinder runner tracks are preferred surfaces. Motorized treadmills offer resilient surface for walking and jogging.

Summary

▶ Preventing exercise-related injuries requires adherence to common sense safety principles.

▶ The R-I-C-E principle represents the general treatment for many types of exercise-related injuries.

▶ Wear quality walking or jogging shoes.

▶ In the beginning, walk or jog every other day and increase the frequency to a level consistent with improvement and program objectives.

▶ Increase frequency and duration of exercise prior to increasing intensity.

▶ Adjust intensity and duration of the workout to accommodate the environmental conditions.

▶ Hydrate fully prior to working out and continue to drink liquid during and after.

▶ Follow sound warm-up and cool-down procedures.

▶ Strive to improve your walking or jogging form.

▶ Choose walking and jogging surfaces that are less likely to produce injuries.

REFERENCES

1. Fahey, T. D., Insel, P. M., and Roth, W. T. *Core Concepts and Labs in Physical Fitness and Wellness*, Mountain View, CA: Mayfield Publishing Co., 1994.

2. Leach, R. E. et al. "Achilles Tendonitis," *The Physician and Sportsmedicine*, 19: (August, 1991), p. 87.

3. Taylor, D. C. et al. "Viscoelastic Properties of Muscle-Tendon Units: The Biomechanical Effects of Stretching," *American Journal of Sports Medicine*, 18, No. 3: (1990), p. 300.

4. Ritter, M. A., and Albohm, M.J. *Your Injury*, Carmel, Indiana: Benchmark Press, Inc., 1987.

5. de Vries, H. A. and Housh, T. J. *Physiology of Exercise*, Madison: WCB Brown and Benchmark, 1994.

6. Williams, M. H. *Lifetime Fitness and Wellness*, Madison: WCB Brown and Benchmark, 1993.

7. Newham, D. J. et al. "Large Delayed Plasma Creatine Kinase Changes After Stepping Exercise," *Muscle Nerve*, 6: (June, 1983), p. 380.

8. Torg, J. S. et al. "Overuse Injuries in Sport: The Foot," *Clinics in Sports Medicine*, 6, No. 2: (April, 1987), p. 921.

9. Andrish, J. and Work, J. A. "How I Manage Shin Splints," *The Physician and Sportsmedicine*, 18, No. 12: (December, 1990), p. 113.

10. Fick, D. S. et al. "Relieving Painful Skin Splints," *The Physician and Sportsmedicine*, 20, No. 12: (December, 1992), p. 105.

11. Chadbourne, R. D. "A Hard Look at Running Surfaces," *The Physician and Sportsmedicine*, 18, No. 7: (July, 1990), p. 102.

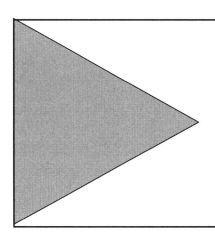

Glossary of Terms

Aerobic exercise   Literally means "with oxygen." It is the ability to supply the oxygen needed for exercise while the individual is exercising.

Allergen   Any substance that produces an allergic response.

Amenorrhea   Cessation of the menstrual cycle.

Anabolism   The assimilation of nutrients and their conversion to living tissue.

Anaerobic exercise   Literally means "without oxygen." Refers to high intensity exercise where the oxygen demand cannot be met during the time that one is exercising.

Android obesity   The masculine pattern of fat deposition in the abdomen, chest, and back.

Asthmogenic   Substances or events that are capable of producing bronchospasms.

Atherosclerosis   A slow progressive disease of large and medium size arteries characterized by the formation of plaque.

Blood plasma   The liquid portion of the blood.

Body composition   The separation and quantification of fat and lean body tissues.

Carcinogenic   Substances that are capable of producing cancer.

Cardiac reserve   HR max minus RHR.

Cardiovascular disease   Disease of the heart and coronary blood vessels.

Catabolism   The breakdown of complex chemical compounds into simpler ones for use by the body.

Catecholamines   Consist of the hormones epinephrine and norepinephrine; they are stimulants to the circulatory system and constrict blood vessels.

Chronic diseases   Long lasting and/or frequently occurring diseases that are genetic or lifestyle induced.

Chronic stress   Long term stress, persistent exposure to a stressor or group of stressors.

Communicable Diseases   Severe diseases of short duration caused by microbes.

Concentric muscle contraction   A muscle that shortens while lifting a weight against the force of gravity.

Coronary heart disease   Disease of the heart caused by atherosclerotic narrowing of the coronary arteries.

Cross-training   A system of training that employs a variety of activities rather than focusing on just one.

Dehydration   Excessive fluid loss from the body.

Depression   Prolonged sadness that persists beyond a reasonable length of time.

Distress   Negative stress.

Dynamic stretching   A system for stretching muscles and joints that involves bouncing and bobbing movements.

Eccentric muscle contraction   A muscle that lengthens resisting the force of gravity while returning the weight to the starting position.

Electrocardiograph (ECG)   An instrument that monitors the electric activity of the heart.

Epinephrine   A hormone secreted by the adrenal glands that constricts blood vessels.

Estrogen   A female sex hormone responsible for the development of secondary sexual characteristics and for various phases of the menstrual cycle.

Eustress   Positive stress.

External (Extrinsic) rewards   Rewards administered by outside sources. These can be symbolic, material or psychological.

Goals   An end or objective to be achieved.

Gynoid obesity   The feminine pattern of fat deposition in the hips, buttocks, and thighs.

Health promotion programs   Include lifestyle behaviors that are conducive to health enhancement, such as, exercise, smoking cessation, blood pressure screening, cholesterol evaluation, stress management, weight control, etc.

Health-related fitness   Type of fitness that emphasizes development of cardiorespiratory endurance, muscular strength and endurance, flexibility, and lean body composition.

Hematocrit   The ratio of red blood cells to plasma volume.

Hemoglobin   Iron pigment of the red blood cells that carries oxygen and carbon dioxide.

Homeostasis   The state of equilibrium in the body with respect to various functions and to the chemical composition of fluids and tissues.

Hyperthermia   Excessive heat accumulation in the body.

Hypothermia   Excessive heat lost from the body.

Inflammation   A diseased condition produced by an infection, injury, or irritant and is characterized by heat, redness, swelling and pain.

Insoluble fiber   Dietary fiber in polysaccharides that is insoluable in hot water. It enhances the health of the intestines by speeding food remnants through them.

Internal (Intrinsic) rewards   Reinforcement coming from within; the degree of satisfaction derived in the absence of some visible reward.

Ischemia   Diminished blood flow.

Kilocalories (kcals)   This represents the number of calories found in food.

Lipid   The scientific term for "fat."

Malignant   Tumors or tissues that are cancerous.

Menopause   The decline and eventual cessation of hormone production by the reproductive system in mid-life; the termination of the menstrual cycle.

Menstruation   The monthly flow of blood from the uterine lining.

Metabolic diseases   This category of diseases includes diabetes mellitus, thyroid disorders, kidney disease, liver disease, and other less common diseases.

Metabolism   The sum of the chemical changes occurring in tissues consisting of anabolism and catabolism.

Morbidity   The sick rate in a population.

Mortality   The death rate in a population.

Motivation   The internal mechanisms and external stimuli that arouse and stimulate behavior.

Myocardial infarction   The medical term for a heart attack.

Myotatic reflex   A proprioceptor in the center of muscles that responds to forceful stretch.

Neoplasm   New tissue or tumor.

Norepinephrine   A hormone secreted by the adrenal glands that constricts blood vessels.

Oncogene   A cancerous gene.

Orthotic   Orthopedic devices placed in shoes designed to correct walking or jogging gaits.

Overfat   Excessive fat: for males 23% to 25% or more of the body weight is fat and females 32% or more of the body weight is fat.

Overweight   Excessive weight for height.

O_2 debt   The amount of O_2 required during recovery from exercise that is over and above that which is normally required at rest.

O_2 deficit   The first one or two minutes of exercise when the O_2 demand exceeds the body's ability to supply it.

Performance-related fitness   The type of fitness that allows one to perform physical skills with a high degree of proficiency.

Positive reinforcement   A reward or action that increases the strength of a response.

R-I-C-E principle   This is an acronym which stands for rest, ice, compression, and elevation of an injured body part.

Risk factors   Genetic tendencies and learned behaviors that increase the probability of premature illness and death.

Soluble Fiber   Dietary fiber in polysaccharides that is soluable in hot water. It adds bulk to the contents of the stomach and lowers serum cholesterol.

Static stretching   A system of stretching where stretch positions are held in a fixed manner for 15 to 30 seconds.

Stressors   Any condition, circumstance, or event that provokes the stress response.

Thrombus   A blood clot.

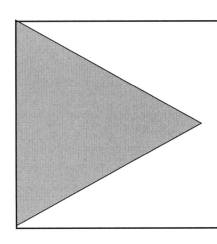

Index